COMMUNITY HOSPITALS AND RURAL ACCESSIBILITY

Community Hospitals and Rural Accessibility

R.M. HAYNES
C.G. BENTHAM

University of East Anglia

assisted by

M.B. SPENCER

Transport Studies Unit,
University of Oxford

and

J.M. SPRATLEY

Department of Community Health,
University of Nottingham

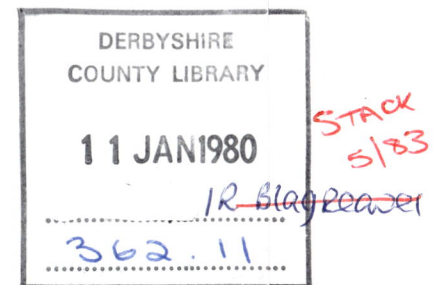
SAXON HOUSE

British Library Cataloguing in Publication Data

Haynes, R M
   Community hospitals and rural accessibility.
   1. Hospitals, Rural - England - King's Lynn region
   2. Hospitals, Rural - England
   I. Title   II. Bentham, C G
   362.1'1   RA988.K/

   ISBN 0-566-00271-X

Published by
Teakfield Limited,
Westmead, Farnborough, Hants., England.

Printed by
Itchen Printers Limited, Southampton

ISBN 0 566 00271 X

Contents

Preface

This book reports the work of the community hospital planning study at
the University of East Anglia from 1976 to 1978. The study explored
the feasibility of implementing the DHSS community hospital policy in
a rural health district and investigated a method for assessing some
of the benefits to the rural community of dispersed hospital services.
It was funded by the Social Science Research Council, whose support
we gratefully acknowledge.

The approach adopted was to examine a particular health district in
detail with the object of drawing general conclusions from it.
We were fortunate throughout in enjoying the cooperation and help of
officers of the King's Lynn Health District, the Norfolk Area Health
Authority and the East Anglian Regional Health Authority. We are
grateful to them for their encouragement and assistance. While their
goodwill was indispensible for our work, neither these people nor the
health authorities they represent are in any way responsible for the
contents of this report. The responsibility is ours alone, as it is
also for any errors that may be found.

We extend our thanks in addition to officers of the Norwich Health
District, the Lincolnshire Area Health Authority, the King's Lynn
Community Health Council, the Lincolnshire North Community Health
Council, the staff of the Wallingford Community Hospital and the staff
of the hospitals where our surveys were conducted. Many individuals
were consulted during the course of the study and we thank them all,
particularly Professor R.M. Acheson, Dr. J.S.A. Ashley, Professor
A.E. Bennett, Professor C.M. Elliott, Professor A.R. Emerson, Dr. M.
Hall-Smith, Dr. T. Heller and Dr. F.C. Rutter. We also wish to record
our gratitude to the hundreds of people who answered our questions and
so provided the information on which this book is based. Finally we
thank our typist, Mrs. J.T. Carr.

1 Introduction

As the hospital service becomes increasingly concentrated in the main
towns and cities, the future of many small hospitals in England and
Wales is in doubt.   Proposals have been made by many health authorities
to close small local hospitals that are thought to be surplus to the
requirements of a modern service but even hints of closure have aroused
considerable local opposition, particularly in rural areas where access
to a district centre may be difficult.   In 1974, the Department of
Health and Social Security put forward its "community hospitals" policy,
which defined a new and useful role for the small hospital as a place
where patients who do not need the specialised facilities of a district
general hospital could be cared for.   All health authorities were
encouraged to develop at least some of their small local hospitals as
"community hospitals".   The work reported here explores the feasibility of the community hospital ideal and investigates some of the costs
and benefits to the rural community of a decentralised hospital system.

ORIGINS OF THE POLICY

The National Health Service inherited a collection of hospitals of
great variety.   The first national hospital plan (Ministry of Health,
1962) took as its priority the gradual replacement of this historically
determined scattering of hospitals by an orderly pattern of district
general hospitals, normally of 600-800 beds and serving a population of
100,000-150,000.   Each district general hospital would concentrate
facilities for diagnosis and treatment on a single site.   The trend
towards centralisation and the emphasis on large hospitals was given
fresh impetus by the Bonham Carter Report (Central Health Services
Council, 1969) which recommended even larger district general hospitals
and the closure of small hospitals in towns within reach of a district
general hospital.   Only in remote areas were "outpost" hospital units
to be encouraged.   Modern scientific advances in medicine and surgery
had been fully matched by rising public expectations with regard to
health care and these could only be met in purpose-built general
hospitals serving a large enough population to justify sophisticated
facilities and full consultant cover.   The building programme is now
well established, although under the financial stringency of the last
few years the latest projects have been scaled down into "nucleus
hospitals", which are still large at about 300 beds and capable of
future expansion.   These improvements command an increasing share of
the resources of all health authorities and many older and smaller
hospitals are being recommended for closure, although actual closure
has often proved to be politically difficult.

Housed, as they are for the most part, in buildings of the last
century, small local hospitals are often inconvenient in structure and
too costly to maintain as high standard acute hospitals.   Yet for all

their faults small hospitals are well supported by their local communities and attract high levels of voluntary involvement as well as dedicated professional service. They also provide advantages for some patients over those of a district general hospital. A positive feature is their friendly and informal atmosphere, which results from both small size and the day to day contacts between staff and other members of the community outside the hospital itself. Especially for elderly patients who might be bewildered and even frightened by the unfamiliar efficiency of a busy general hospital, a more homely environment and the reassurance of having their own general practitioner at hand is to be preferred. Many small hospitals are run by local general practitioners and can provide a continuity of care much needed by some patients. Then there are the more direct benefits of accessibility. A hospital with a limited local catchment area involves much less travel on the part of the patient and his visitors, so that family life is less disrupted than it would be by admission to a larger and consequently more distant hospital.

These advantages are perhaps only marginal ones for the majority of hospital patients, who are admitted for a short episode while acutely ill or to undergo surgery. Such patients require above all a specialised level of skill and facilities, which are the services the district general hospital is designed to supply. But not all hospital patients fall into this category. Many elderly people, the chronically sick and physically and mentally handicapped people are also to be found in hospitals, not so much because they require sophisticated investigations or treatment but because they need longer term nursing or rehabilitative support which cannot be provided at home. These people for whom a bed in a district general hospital would be unnecessarily expensive are the very patients who would be expected to benefit from the more homely atmosphere and accessibility of the small local hospital.

For elderly people in particular, hospital beds are expected to be subject to growing demand as the proportion of elderly persons in the population continues to increase over the next ten years. This is a serious short term problem which small local hospitals could help to alleviate. Because of relatively low birth rates during the interwar period, a decline in the proportion of elderly people is forecast for the 1990s (Central Statistical Office, 1977).

Local hospitals might also help to ease the pressure on acute beds in the district general hospital by accepting patients who have already received the most intensive part of their treatment but who are not yet ready to return home. Furthermore, many patients not at present in hospital but being looked after by their families at home might benefit from a short period of rehabilitation in a local hospital that would prolong their lives in the community and obviate or delay their eventual admission as long term in-patients. For the families of such patients, a short period of admission would temporarily ease the burden, perhaps enabling them to take a holiday. Other people who could benefit from physiotherapy, occupational therapy or other remedial treatment might be given the opportunity to receive these services regularly in a day ward of a local hospital, returning to their homes in the evening. By being a focus of health care at the local level, the small hospital might help to foster greater contact and coordination between the health and social services and also between those services and the public, so facilitating early diagnosis and treatment.

The district general hospital is unsuitable for this role because it is too large and remote : familiarity and accessibility are key conditions.

Used in this way, small local hospitals would provide a complementary service, rather than being just miniature and relatively inefficient replicas of the district general hospital. They would supply a much needed link in between the general hospital service and the community. They could, indeed, be regarded as extensions of primary care, to help families, general practitioners and the various domiciliary services to look after patients more effectively at home and maybe in the long term reduce the demand for acute hospital beds.

It was in this spirit that the first "community hospital" experiments were initiated in the late 1960s by the Oxford Regional Hospital Board. In 1969 the Norman White Ward at the Peppard Hospital (near Reading and originally a chest hospital) was reopened as a community hospital ward available for use by local general practitioners. The ward consisted of 15 beds, a treatment room, dining room and offices. A day ward was added later. Following the success of this pilot trial, the first purpose-designed community hospital was opened in Wallingford in 1973 to serve the town of Wallingford and its surrounding villages (Bennett, 1974).

The core of the Wallingford Community Hospital is a health centre which is the focal point of all the primary health care activities in the locality. It accommodates the surgeries of a partnership of five general practitioners and the offices of the district nurses, midwives and health visitors. It has a treatment room and pathological specimen collecting facilities. Accommodation is also provided for peripheral consultant clinics in a wide range of specialties and for local authority clinics such as ante natal and dental clinics and clinics in speech therapy, child health, health education and hearing assessment, to name a few. For patients who need remedial support and who are able to return to their homes at night there is a day unit with 20 places, staffed by physiotherapists and occupational therapists. Finally, there are the wards for in-patients, originally a 17 bed general ward and a 17 bed maternity ward, later extended to a total of 72 beds. The general ward beds are used for acutely ill people admitted for nursing care that cannot be given at home, patients transferred from district general hospital beds, selected post assessment geriatric and psychiatric patients, selected physically and mentally handicapped patients requiring hospital care, holiday admissions and selected terminal care patients.

The DHSS guidelines for the development of small local hospitals had many points in common with the Wallingford Community Hospital. While there were differences - the official recommendations did not include maternity provision, for example, and placed much more emphasis on beds for geriatric and elderly mentally infirm patients - the community hospital policy clearly owed its development to the Oxford experiments.

THE DHSS GUIDELINES

The Department of Health and Social Security circular on the role and development of community hospitals in the National Health Service appeared in August, 1974. The circular was addressed to all health authorities in England and Wales and made it clear that while many local hospitals would need to be closed as progress was made with the provision of district general hospitals, some existing hospitals that did not form part of the district general hospital scheme might be retained as "community hospitals". Community hospitals were defined as providing medical and nursing care, including out-patient, day patient and in-patient care, for people who do not need the specialised facilities of the district general hospital and cannot be properly cared for at home or in residential accommodation.

The patients considered most suitable for beds in community hospitals were geriatric patients after assessment who no longer require direct access to full diagnostic and treatment facilities, elderly mentally infirm patients needing hospital care and a third group, of medical and surgical patients not in need of the full diagnostic and specialist facilities of the district general hospital. This third category included preconvalescent patients transferred from the district general hospital after completing the most intensive part of their treatment, people with terminal illness who cannot adequately be cared for at home and people with chronic disabilities who need nursing care while their families who normally look after them are on holiday or ill. Specifically excluded from community hospitals were mentally handicapped and mentally ill patients (with the exception of the elderly mentally infirm). It was recommended that maternity patients and children would not normally be included. While patients suffering from minor injuries might be treated in community hospitals, those with other injuries should be taken direct to the accident and emergency unit in the district general hospital. Similarly, any surgical procedures undertaken in community hospitals were recommended not to extend beyond those which general practitioners would expect to perform in their own practice premises or in a health centre. Facilities for general anaesthesia should be provided only for these minor surgical procedures or for dentistry. Limited radiographic services requiring only simple equipment might be needed and the pathology service should be limited to specimen collection, for analysis elsewhere.

It was expected that the day to day care of patients in community hospitals would be the responsibility of general practitioners, working in co-operation with the appropriate consultants. Where possible, health centres and other group practice premises should be closely associated with the hospital, preferably on the same site. While the district general hospital would be the main point to which patients were referred for specialist assessment advice and treatment, it was intended that consultants should hold appropriate out-patient clinics at community hospitals. Physiotherapists and occupational therapists were regarded as essential for the community hospital, for remedial work with both day patients and in-patients. A 24 hour nursing service would, of course, be required.

On the question of the scale of provision, the circular explicitly stated that the introduction of community hospitals should not increase the total number of beds planned to be provided per thousand population. Indeed, it was expected that in many districts fewer beds per thousand population might be needed in the future as the primary health care services develop, local authority residential homes are improved and lengths of stay in district general hospitals are reduced. The guidelines were that community hospitals might provide up to half the geriatric beds and most of the beds for elderly persons suffering from dementia needed for the population served, that is up to 10 beds per 10,000 population. They might also provide up to one fifth of the medical and surgical beds for their population, that is up to 5 beds per 10,000 population served. Overall, then, up to 15 beds per 10,000 population might be in community hospitals. The recommended size for a community hospital was between 50 and 150 beds, a size, incidentally, that more than one third of all existing hospitals in England fail to meet (DHSS, 1977a). Up to half the geriatric day places required for the population and all the day places for elderly mentally infirm persons could be provided in community hospitals. Together this amounts to up to 4 places per 1,000 of the elderly population of the catchment area. Community hospitals might also provide a "considerable number" of out-patient clinics.

In rural areas, it was recommended that community hospitals should be sited in towns which are economic and social centres for the surrounding population. Accessibility and convenience for patients and their relatives were stressed as important factors in determining where community hospitals should be located and a study of communications was suggested to be an essential prerequisite in choosing a site. The availability of staff was also identified as a critical factor when deciding locations, including the willingness of general practitioners who live near the hospital to devote time to working in it. Authorities were asked to ensure that community hospitals were planned so that they did not deplete the district general hospital of scarce staff, particularly nursing staff. For the most part, community hospitals were expected to depend on staff already living in the locality, including staff who would not otherwise be available to the service but who might be attracted to working in the local hospital by its nearness to their homes.

The circular proposed that health authorities should provide community hospitals both by conversion of existing hospitals and by new building. The existing hospitals which might be adapted must be sited where they would be needed and must be of sufficient size or capable of being extended. Many existing hospitals were considered unlikely to be suitable. The provision of community hospitals was to be a long term aim, but health authorities were requested to begin the task of deciding how many would be needed to serve each district, how they should be provided and where they should be sited. The DHSS was at pains to point out that there was room in the policy for local flexibility. Not all community hospitals should have exactly the same functions or operate in the same way, but the guidelines should be adapted to meet local circumstances and needs.

Since 1974, the Department's view has been modified somewhat. The latest strategy statement appeared in a September 1977 publication on priorities in the Health and Social Services: "The Way Forward"

(DHSS, 1977b). In this document the community hospital policy was broadly confirmed but development was stated as being likely to be slower than originally hoped because of financial restrictions, especially in the capital programme. Although the possibility of providing new buildings was included in 1974, it seems that the policy must for the present be interpreted almost entirely in terms of guiding the adaptation of existing local hospitals and helping to determine which existing hospitals are to survive. In the 1977 document the definition of a community hospital was significantly widened to include any retained local hospital which is not part of a district general hospital service. Health authorities were encouraged to "develop community hospitals to provide effectively, among other services, rehabilitation and continuing care of elderly patients, including elderly severely mentally infirm ", but advised that the detailed guidelines given in the original circular "should not stand in the way of flexible and practical solutions agreed locally" (DHSS, 1977b).

POLICY ISSUES

A question which immediately arises is to what extent are practical local solutions likely to diverge from the 1974 ideal? Is the network of community hospitals as seen by the DHSS in 1974 an attainable goal for a typical rural health district? If community hospitals or some local version of them are feasible, how should the health authority go about its task of deciding how many would be needed for each district, how they should be provided and where they should be sited? Although the purpose of this book is to provide information that will help to answer some of these questions, we recognise from the outset that a full evaluation of the community hospital policy is beyond our scope. Particularly difficult issues are the fundamental ones of the medical benefits and the overall costs of community hospital care compared with the alternatives of district general hospital or domiciliary care. Some progress with these issues has been made by the Health Services Evaluation Group in Oxford (Bennett, 1974; Rickard, 1976).

Whether patients benefit medically from the community hospital system and whether these patients are more satisfied can only be tested by a random allocation experiment in which patients deemed suitable for community hospital treatment are assigned randomly either to a district general hospital or a community hospital and their subsequent progress is monitored. This type of experiment, which was conducted in the Oxford Region with the consent of patients, has the appearance of elegance, but is fraught with problems of interpretation. For example, if patients discharged from one type of hospital are found to receive more home visits from their general practitioner and district nurse than those from the other hospital, does this mean that their treatment has been less successful or that the hospital has succeeded in getting them back into the community at an earlier stage? The question of cost is also deceptive. In normal circumstances the cost of maintaining a general hospital bed is likely to be more than the cost for a community hospital bed (the fact that this was found not to be the case in the Oxford pilot trial can be ascribed to an unusually favourable staffing ratio), but the issue is wider than this. Because community hospitals are intended to work in conjunction with other types of primary care their costing must take account of the additional demands on the

6

domiciliary activities of general practitioners, district nurses, social workers, Meals on Wheels, and so on. It can also be argued that some of the really important costs are non-monetary and external ones, since the burden of caring falls on families for the most part, and this burden is relieved only temporarily by the National Health Service. Staff satisfaction is yet another element of the problem. What will be the consequences in the general hospital when all the "easy" cases are removed?

Another fundamental and thorny question concerns the overall scale of provision and the level of health care "need" in the community. The DHSS recommends that up to a quarter of a district total hospital beds may be of the community hospital type; that is, up to 15 beds per 10,000 population, but is this the best ratio? The recommendation is based on present bed ratios, but perhaps not all patients in hospital ought to be there on strictly medical grounds and, conversely, some people not in hospital may be more ill or more dependent than a proportion of hospital patients. How many community hospital beds, then, does the population ideally need? The answer, of course, is that the question is misconceived. Demand for community hospital beds might be expected to keep pace with almost any practicable level of supply. The population will always "need" a few more beds than the number supplied. As the level of provision is ultimately dependent on the amount of public funds available, the question of health care needs is a political not a medical one. The best level of community hospital provision must be decided not by academic study but by political debate.

There are other fundamental questions, however, that offer more hope of yielding to academic investigation. One is the problem of assessing the social costs of a particular hospital plan. A proposal to develop a certain number of community hospitals in a health district, for example, will not only have implications for National Health Service spending but also less obvious implications in terms of the costs that will be borne directly by the community at large. These will include the monetary costs of travel to the hospitals as well as non-monetary costs such as serious inconvenience or even the cost of not being able to reach the hospital at all. Hitherto it has been easier for health authorities to estimate their own costs than to assess the consequences of their decisions to the community. This study will attempt to redress the balance by providing information on some of the costs to the community of health authority planning. It will also be concerned with the feasibility of the community hospital policy and how to put the policy into operation.

In practice, the number of community hospitals in a health district, their size and their location will be subject to a number of constraints. The importance of a study of communications and daily travel activities has already been mentioned, for the pattern of market towns and important villages and the geographical extent of their influence will define the maximum number of locations which already exist as communication centres. For the short term at least, the number and location of existing hospital buildings and sites will be another significant limiting factor. Not all these sites can necessarily be used as cost considerations will almost certainly limit the number of community hospitals by setting a lower limit on size. The DHSS has recommended that the lower limit should be 50 beds. If this recommendation is followed, over one third of existing hospitals would be automatically disqualified as they now stand. To find out what room there may be for manoeuvre around the lower size limit, it would be useful to investigate what is known about the relationship between average costs and size for small hospitals.

If running costs may constrain the lower size limit of community hospitals, the upper limit is likely to be set by the organisation and availability of staff, particularly general practitioners. A guide to the maximum radius of travel expected of GPs can only be achieved by questioning a sample of them. As it is desirable for all participating general practitioners to be equally involved (the emergence of "hospital specialist" GPs is counter to the spirit of the policy) perhaps the upper bed limit will be defined by the maximum number of GPs which can successfully constitute a working team. By no means all the GPs in a district are expected to wish to participate, however, and health authorities have no power of compulsion. A survey is therefore required to establish the attitudes of GPs in a rural area to the idea of working in a community hospital. The views of general practitioners will be invaluable in determining whether the most pressing health care problems in a rural area are considered to be those which the community hospital policy was designed to alleviate. Their views are also of interest on the extent to which the functions and facilities of small local hospitals should be modelled on the detailed DHSS guidelines. A parallel survey of the views of hospital doctors should give an idea of the level of agreement or conflict anticipated over the functions of community hospitals. Consultants could also be asked to comment on the scale at which the decentralisation of out-patient clinics might be attempted and the number of in-patients in the present hospital system who would be suitable for care in a community hospital. This last question is necessary to clarify whether the development of community hospitals will immediately take some pressure away from district general hospital beds or whether community hospitals will tend to generate a new demand.

Other key groups of staff are nurses, physiotherapists, occupational therapists and radiographers. To what extent are they likely to be attracted by the idea of working in small hospitals, which may have a relaxed atmosphere, but which will almost certainly offer limited professional scope when compared with a district general hospital? How big a reservoir of trained staff might a market town be expected to possess? How far might these people be expected to travel to work? Could employment in a community hospital actually produce migration into the vicinity? It is hoped that answers to some of these questions will be provided by a survey of the travel patterns, migrational characteristics and attitudes towards their work of the key groups of personnel.

While detailed predictions of likely community hospital costs are perhaps best left to health service accountants, it will be necessary to comment on the implications to the ambulance service of different geographical arrangements of community hospitals. From the community's point of view there is no doubt that a concentrated hospital service is more expensive than a dispersed one, especially in rural areas. But again, the magnitude of the difference needs to be known before public resources are committed over the long term. This entails a study of the costs and other inconveniences which out-patients, in-patients and their visitors are incurring at present. To avoid the bias which may arise from selecting only those people who successfully reach hospital, a study of the mobility characteristics of the population as a whole is also necessary. As the effects of distance will be felt much more acutely by people who are reliant on public transport, it is of interest to know the level of car availability for medical trips amongst disadvantaged groups like the elderly. Distance to a hospital has an effect on the community not only in terms of the costs of over-coming it, for sometimes it may not be overcome at all. The narrowing of opportunities because of inaccessibility is most manifest in the sparsely populated areas of upland Britain but it may also be a problem in the rural areas of central and southern England. An investigation needs to be made to find out whether hospital admission frequencies and out-patient clinic attendances are lower for people who live at greater distances from hospitals than for those who live closer. The diminution of visiting rates with distance is another topic about which not enough is yet known for planning purposes. A survey of a sample of hospital visitors concentrating on trip lengths, modes, costs and other inconveniences might expose the relationship if one exists.

Finally, it would be useful to demonstrate that it is possible to integrate some of the findings of this study in a method to predict the most significant travel implications to patients and visitors of different geographical arrangements of community hospital facilities in a rural district. In keeping with the new flexibility of the policy, it would be most appropriate to be able to do this separately for the various components of the community hospital: consultant out-patient clinics, local authority clinics, health centre, day patients, geriatric in-patients, elderly mentally infirm in-patients and preconvalescent and other in-patients. The most suitable arrangements for provision of each one of these services might then be assembled to produce a system of community hospital facilities that match the particular local circumstances under consideration. To keep the work within manageable bounds, this will be attempted for just four of the components: out-patient clinics and the three main groups of in-patients, although the method should be capable of dealing with the other components as well. When the advantages and disadvantages of various alternative ways of arranging community hospital services in a health district are debated, it would be desirable for estimates of their implications for the community to be set alongside the estimates of cost to the health authority. The aim of the exercise will be to explore a method for arriving at the community estimates.

We have concentrated on describing the planning issues for community hospitals in rural areas rather than urban areas because it is the accessibility problems of the rural setting that the policy appears designed to meet. We have emphasised the types of issue and will endeavour to draw the kinds of conclusion that will be applicable to any rural health district in England and Wales. But a national study is far beyond our scope. Instead, a case study approach is adopted, in which a particular health district is examined for illustrative purposes. The object is not to plan the community hospital facilities of that particular district - that is the function of the area and regional health authorities - but rather to draw general conclusions relevant to community hospital planning from it. The study area chosen is the King's Lynn Health District, which is administered by the

Norfolk Area Health Authority within the East Anglian Region. This
health district is centred on the town of King's Lynn in West Norfolk,
where a new general hospital to serve the acute medical and surgical
needs of the district's population is under construction. The district
is a rural one and contains a number of market towns and a number of
small hospitals.

The study district, its hospitals, communications and the transport
characteristics of its population are described in the next chapter.
Chapter 3 describes questionnaire surveys of doctors and other health
service staff and considers questions of hospital costs, in order to
reach conclusions about the feasibility and functions of rural community
hospitals. In Chapter 4, the costs to patients and visitors in getting
to hospital are investigated, again using questionnaire surveys, and
Chapter 5 discusses the evidence that some trips to hospital by
potential patients and visitors are not being made because of the
difficulties in overcoming distance. A method for estimating the
implications of different community hospital locations for patients
and their visitors is described and its results presented in Chapter 6.
The concluding chapter discusses some of the main findings and their
application elsewhere in rural England and Wales.

2 Hospitals and accessibility in a rural district

This chapter begins with a description of some of the principal
features of the distribution of population in the King's Lynn Health
District and the ways in which that population is changing. It then
goes on to describe the existing hospital services of the district and
the proposals for change following the opening of a new district
general hospital in 1980. Following this introduction to the population of the study district and the hospitals that serve it, the bulk
of the chapter is devoted to a consideration of the transport system
that forms the essential link between the two.

It is becoming widely recognised that the availability of a private
car acts as an extremely important influence on the ease with which
rural dwellers can reach many important services, including hospitals.
Therefore, some of the key issues considered are the way in which car
ownership and availability vary geographically over the King's Lynn
Health District and between different groups in the population. The
ways in which they are likely to change in the future are also discussed.

For those without the use of a car, public transport in rural areas
assumes particular significance. The chapter goes on to discuss some
of the characteristics of the public transport system of the study area
which affect its ability to offer acceptable standards of accessibility
to hospitals. Finally, some aspects of the ambulance service and
hospital car service are considered.

THE POPULATION AND HOSPITALS OF THE KING'S LYNN DISTRICT

The study area, the King's Lynn Health District, is one of the three
districts within the Norfolk Area Health Authority. It comprises
the western part of the county of Norfolk and a smaller part of northern Cambridgeshire around the town of Wisbech (Figure 2.1).

At the time of the last population census in 1971 the population of
the district was approximately 161,000, and the latest (1977) estimate
is 168,000. This population is predominantly rural with 63% of the
total living outside the towns. The rural character of the area is
further emphasised by the low population density of 0.77 persons per
hectare.

King's Lynn is the largest town in the district (Table 2.1). It is
a port and has a substantial amount of manufacturing industry. One of
its major functions is to act as the main shopping, business and
service centre for most of west Norfolk.

Wisbech, a town which is a little more than half the size of King's
Lynn, provides a similar range of services to a smaller area in the
western part of the district. Below the level of these two main towns

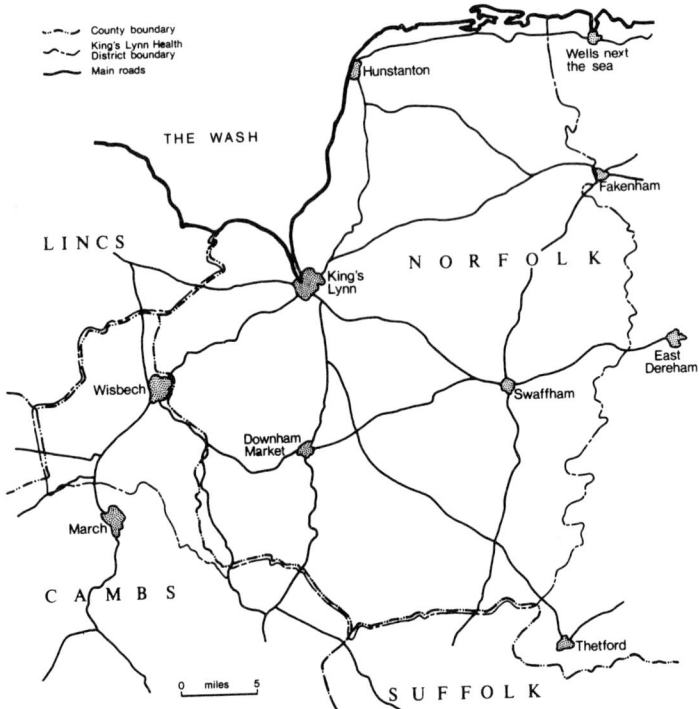

Figure 2.1   The King's Lynn Health District

Table 2.1
Population in 1971

King's Lynn M.B.	30,100
Wisbech M.B.	17,000
Swaffham U.D.	4,300
Downham Market U.D.	3,600
Hunstanton U.D.	3,900
Remainder of the Health District	101,800
	160,700

the area is little urbanised.   Swaffham and Downham Market are small
market towns which serve their surrounding areas.   The only other town
is Hunstanton which is primarily a small holiday resort.   The remainder
of the population of the district live in a variety of different types
of rural settlement.

At one extreme are the commuter villages, around the two main towns,
particularly King's Lynn.   These are often fairly large, accessible to
the services offered by the towns, recently developed and with a young
and moderately affluent population.   At the other extreme there are
parts of north and central Norfolk which are much more traditionally
rural: inaccessible and sparsely populated, with a declining and age-
ing population.

Like the rest of Norfolk, the population of the district has been growing in recent years and the latest estimates are that this growth will continue in the future, albeit at a slower rate (Table 2.2). Although there are no figures specifically for the district, it is likely that in-migration has been a more important contributor to this growth than natural increase. For the county as a whole migration has accounted for about two-thirds of total increase. Some of this has been planned migration, for example, the movement of overspill population into King's Lynn as part of a Town Development Scheme. There has also been much non-planned migration, much of it of young families, but also with a significant number of retired people.

Table 2.2
Population projections for the district

1971	1977	1981	1986	1991
160,700	168,000	173,700	177,800	182,400

Source: East Anglian Regional Health Authority (1977)

The age structure of the population has also been changing with a tendency for the proportion of old people to increase. By 1974, people of retirement age accounted for about 20% of the total population of the county, compared with 17% in 1961. For the King's Lynn District it is anticipated that the percentage of the population aged 65 and over will remain constant at 17% until 1991, although the proportion of people older than 75 is expected to increase (East Anglian Regional Health Authority, 1977).

However, these total figures mask substantial differences between different parts of the district. King's Lynn and the commuter villages around it have been growing quite rapidy. King's Lynn itself has received overspill population (340 persons per annum during the period 1966-75) as part of the Town Development Scheme, whilst during the same period spontaneous growth in the King's Lynn area has been even greater (Norfolk County Council, 1977). Associated with these trends is the tendency towards there being more young people in the population of the King's Lynn area. This contrasts with rural depopulation, particularly in the remote northern parts of Norfolk, during the 1960s, continuing in a few areas into the 1970s. Since out-migration is predominantly of younger, more skilled, people this has produced an ageing population in such areas, a tendency accentuated by retirement migration into some of the coastal villages. One result of these trends is a concentration of large proportions of the elderly in some of the remoter parts of the district. Another result is relatively high proportions of the less skilled in such areas.

There are at present twelve hospitals in the district providing a total of 830 beds. These range in size from the 162 bed West Norfolk and King's Lynn General Hospital to the 18 bed Swaffham Cottage Hospital. The beds are overwhelmingly concentrated in the two main towns. King's Lynn has 480 and Wisbech 256, with the whole of the remainder of the district having only 94. The main acute hospitals for the district are the West Norfolk and King's Lynn General Hospital, and the smaller North Cambridgeshire Hospital in Wisbech. Provision for geriatric patients is in the St. James' Hospital in King's Lynn and the Clarkson Hospital in Wisbech. The sizes and functions of the other hospitals are summarised in Table 2.3, which is based on the Norfolk Area Health Authority's Consultation Paper on the hospital services of the district (Norfolk Area Health Authority, 1978).

Table 2.3
The hospitals in the King's Lynn district

Hospital	Classification	No. of beds	Remarks
In King's Lynn			
West Norfolk & King's Lynn General Hospital	Acute	162	Overcrowded,inadequate and obsolete.
The Windsor Unit	Adult Mental Handicap	48	Opened in 1971
St. James' Hospital	Mainly long stay (Geriatric) but including 20 post-operative ortho-paedic beds	140	By any standards sprawling,incredibly inconvenient for nursing purposes,expensive to maintain and increasingly a structural liability.
Chatterton House	Mental illness	30	The pressure on this small unit for the treatment of psychiatric patients is already greater than it can conveniently carry
The Hardwick Hospital	Chest and isolation	26	A well run unit. The building,difficult of access from a main traffic route and adjacent to a cemetery, has nothing to recommend its retention
The Queen Elizabeth Maternity Department	Maternity	74	A modern unit opened in 1971 as the first phase of new hospital provision

14

Table 2.3 continued

Hospital	Classification	No. of beds	Remarks
In Wisbech			
North Cambridge-shire Hospital	Acute	91	The medical wards,out-patient departments and operating theatre are of excellent modern standard while the surgical wards urgently require radical up-grading.
The Clarkson Hospital	Mainly long stay	123	This ex-public assist-ance institution,while well adapted,can never provide an adequate standard of accommo-dation. A modern associated day hospital was opened in 1976.
The Bowthorpe Maternity Hospital	Maternity	42	An excellent unit, extensively modernised in 1967. However,the new district general hospital will be more than sufficient to carry the full obstet-ric work load of the district.
Elsewhere			
Hunstanton Recovery Hospital (in Hunstanton)	Convalescent	36	Well situated on the sea front,but struct-ural limitations restrict it to conval-escent patients and preclude development as a rehabilitation unit.
Stow Hall Hospital (3 miles north Downham Market)	Preconvalescent	40	Distant from the general hospital in King's Lynn and with poor clinical amenit-ies. Rented by the Health Service. Its use has been necessary rather than convenient.

Table 2.3 continued

Hospital	Classification	No. of beds	Remarks
Swaffham Cottage Hospital (in Swaffham)	Acute	18	The general practitioner staff admit patients who would require a bed in some other unit if this hospital were not available.

Virtually all the district's out-patient clinics are held in either King's Lynn (about two thirds) or Wisbech (about one third). In King's Lynn the largest number of clinic sessions is held at the West Norfolk and King's Lynn General Hospital, although clinics are also held at St. James' Hospital. In Wisbech the North Cambridgeshire Hospital is the main venue, although the Bowthorpe Maternity Hospital also holds clinics.

In several respects the present provision of hospital services in the King's Lynn Health District is recognised as inadequate. The remarks taken from the Area Health Authority's consultation paper in Table 2.3 make it plain that while all hospitals are at present performing necessary functions, their long term futures are open to question. The same consultation paper also compares the provision of beds in the main specialties with the number of beds indicated by the district's projected 1981 population when national norms are applied. Only obstetrics and paediatrics have more hospital beds than the population would appear to warrant and the following specialties are under-provided to the extent of 30-90 beds each (in decreasing order): elderly mentally infirm, mental handicap, geriatrics, mental illness, general medicine and general surgery. The worst under-provision is for the elderly and the mentally ill and handicapped. Although the district could justify 87 beds for the elderly mentally infirm on the basis of the norm of three beds per thousand population aged 65 or over, at present there are no beds within the district for such patients.

In recognition of the deficiencies of the hospital provision in the district the Department of Health and Social Security has sanctioned the construction of a new district general hospital of the "best buy" pattern. This is currently being built on a site on the out-skirts of King's Lynn. When opened in 1980, it will provide 521 beds (see Table 2.4) and will produce a radical change in the hospital services of the district. The implications will go far beyond the new facilities in the district general hospital itself. On current estimates (at 1975/76 prices) the district general hospital will have revenue costs of £4,216,000 out of a district total for hospital services of £5,623,000, thus leaving £1,347,000 for all the remaining hospitals (Norfolk Area Health Authority, 1978). This new situation clearly implies the closure or alteration of function of the existing hospitals in the district.

Table 2.4
Beds in the new district general hospital

Speciality	Beds
General medicine, including chest	92
Paediatrics	28
General surgery	72
Orthopaedics	68
E.N.T.	19
Day/Emergency Ward	20
Ophthamology	11
Dental	3
Gynaecology and Obstetrics	102
Special Care babies	20
Geriatrics	86

At the time of writing, the topic is still one of debate and public controversy. What does seem clear is that the new district general hospital will take over most of the functions of the obsolete West Norfolk and King's Lynn General Hospital, which could then be developed as a geriatric unit, and at least some of the acute functions of the North Cambridgeshire Hospital, which might then accommodate an increasing proportion of the community hospital type of patient. Some community hospital functions might also be provided by the Bowthorpe Maternity Hospital (if its present role is entirely taken over by the district general hospital), Swaffham Cottage Hospital and, for the short term, Stow Hall Hospital near Downham Market and the Clarkson Hospital in Wisbech. It is emphasised that these are not necessarily the strategies advocated by the Norfolk Area Health Authority, nor are they representative of the proposals of the more prominent public pressure groups in the district. What these suggestions do show, however, is that the opportunity exists in the King's Lynn District to develop a hospital system consisting of a new district general hospital and a number of smaller units with community hospital functions.

CAR OWNERSHIP AND AVAILABILITY

Having outlined some of the salient features of the population of the district and the distribution of hospital facilities within it, the remainder of this chapter is devoted to a more detailed discussion of the principal factors determining the accessibility of these facilities to the population. This section considers private car transport and the sections following deal with public transport and health service transport.

The single most important factor in determining the mobility enjoyed by an individual living in a rural area is the extent to which a private car is available for his or her use. Car availability is not synonymous with car ownership since one or two members of a car owning household may have almost exclusive use of the vehicle, particularly at certain times of day. However, more is known about car ownership

than car availability and it is appropriate to begin a study of
mobility with some discussion of this factor.

Car ownership

Car ownership levels are high in East Anglia. Table 2.5 shows the
proportions of households with one, two or more cars in that region
compare with similar proportions in the much more affluent regions of
the southeast and southwest, and outstrip the rates in the remainder of
Great Britain.

The dispersed and rural character of settlement in East Anglia has
undoubtedly contributed to the region's position in the list. Rural
areas generally have higher levels of car ownership than urban areas
because of the greater trip lengths involved in reaching jobs, shops
and other facilities. Areas of low population density are associated
with high car ownership levels (Fishwick, 1972; Rhys and Buxton,1974).
Rural areas also have poorer public transport than urban areas, and
public transport provision is also significant in explaining variations
in car ownership (Fairhurst, 1975; Edwards, 1977).

Table 2.5
Percentage of households with regular use of a car 1974-5

Percentage of households with:	2+ cars	1 car	No car
Southwest	14	55	31
Southeast	17	49	34
East Anglia	12	54	34
West Midlands	12	47	40
East Midlands	11	48	41
Wales	9	50	41
North	7	45	48
Northwest	8	41	50
Yorkshire and Humberside	7	43	50
Greater London	8	41	50
Scotland	6	40	54

Source: Department of Transport (1977)

At the local level the principal source of car ownership information
is the census, the latest available figures being for 1971. Car
ownership information for the parishes of the King's Lynn Health
District taken from the 1971 census is shown in Figure 2.2. The parishes
picked out on the map are those with relatively high and low proportions
of households with one or more cars. No clear pattern is apparent
except for the cluster of parishes in the north with low car ownership.

A similar map of the proportion of households owning two or more
cars suggests the same spatial pattern. In order to explain the
variations in car ownership between parishes it is necessary to
examine not only the quality of public transport and the density of

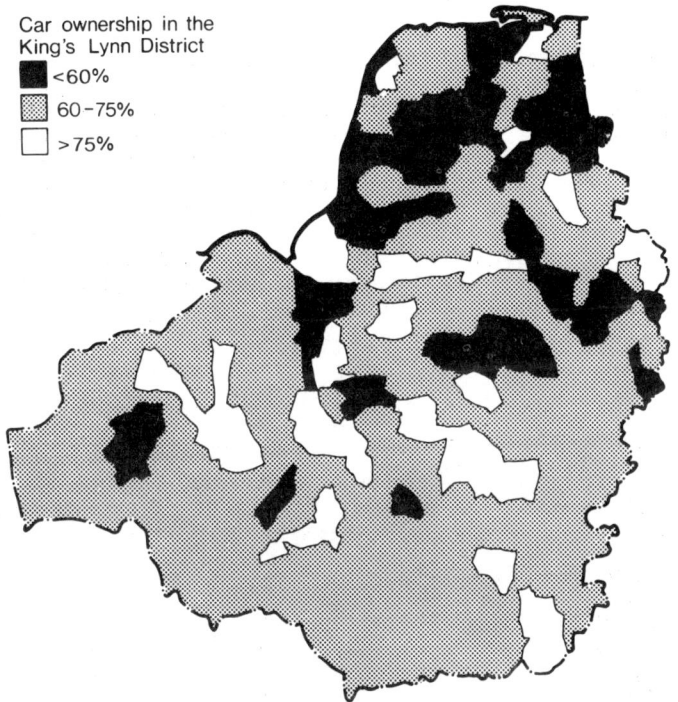

Car ownership in the
King's Lynn District
■ <60%
▨ 60-75%
☐ >75%

Figure 2.2   Car ownership

land use in the locality but also the socio-economic characteristics
of households in each parish.   Much of the variation in car ownership between households is attributable to household income, as is
demonstrated in Table 2.6.   The information in this table comes
from a rural transport survey of 634 households in 16 rural parishes
in central and northeast Norfolk during 1975 (Moseley et al, 1977a and
b) and is the most recent local source.   Apart from the obvious
increase in car ownership with household income, Table 2.6 shows that
even though the majority of households in the two lowest income groups
did not own a car, the proportion that did manage to purchase and run
a vehicle is surprisingly high.

Car ownership is also related to the ages of the members of households.   The elderly households in the Norfolk rural transport survey
(households consisting entirely of persons of retirement age) were less
likely than younger households to own a car: 65% of elderly households
did not own a car compared with the overall average of 27%.   It is
also true that these households had lower levels of income: 55% of
elderly households reported an annual income of less than £1,000 and
75% had an annual income of below £2,000.   Households containing
elderly people tended also to be smaller.   The fact that all these
influences came together in this type of household illustrates one of
the problems of considering car ownership in a one-dimensional way
(that is, using simply income or age to explain variations in car
ownership).   Relevant factors such as household income, household
size, age of members of the household, socio-economic group and
intangibles such as preferences, values and expectations, are not

independent but are linked together. There is an obvious relationship between household size, the number of economically active members and household income. This, in turn, will be related to the stage in life of the household (a young family with school-age children becomes a family with working sons or daughters, then a working couple with no resident children, and so on). Income and social status are also related to the housing, workplace and service density in the resident-ial area, which is itself connected with car ownership. Whether car ownership is a pre-requisite or a result of residential characteristics does not matter here; car ownership is just one component in a tangled web of relationships.

Table 2.6
Household income by car ownership

1975 Annual income	Percentage of households owning:		
	No cars	1 car	2 or more cars
- £1,000	78	20	2
- £1,500	45	52	3
- £2,000	14	79	7
- £2,500	5	74	21
- £3,000	0	67	23
- £4,000	5	49	46
- £6,000	6	48	46
more than £6,000	0	24	76
All income groups	27	52	21

Source: Moseley et al (1977b)

Forecasting car ownership

Since the 1971 census, the most up to date estimate of car ownership on a regional scale is provided by the National Travel Survey (Department of the Environment, 1976a). For East Anglia as a whole, these estimates suggest a rise from 49% to 54% in the proportion of households owning one car, from 11% to 12% in those owning more than one car and a corresponding fall from 39% to 34% of non car owning households from the census in 1971 to 1974-5. The King's Lynn District had 49% of households with one car and 15% with more than one car in 1971, so on the basis of the regional trend it seems safe to estimate that at least 70% of the district's households own one or more cars at the present time. The rate of increase expected in the future is heavily dependent on the estimate that is made of the eventual saturation level or upper limit.

There is at present no concensus about the saturation level of car ownership (estimates range from 0.3 to 0.66 cars per person and the official forecasts are based upon a saturation point of 0.45 cars per person). The official forecasts have been heavily criticised (Depart-ment of Transport, 1978). In general, these forecasts are elaborate ways of projecting past trends and do not add to our understanding of the decision-making process which individuals and households adopt in

20

relation to car ownership. Locally, in areas like Norfolk, it is possible that the saturation level of 0.45 cars per person used in the official forecasts will be exceeded as a result of the greater incentives that exist in rural areas for car ownership and the migration of car owning households. The gradual replacement of car-less by car owning households might be hastened by the continued decline in conventional public transport and the changing age structure of some rural areas. The pattern of migration is therefore important in determining the spatial variation in car ownership in the future. The deeper rural areas may be avoided by the younger economically active, who may predominate in the commuter hinterlands of the employment centres. The more remote areas may continue to attract a small number of retirement migrants who are less likely to own cars, particularly as they age.

Car availability

From surveys of eastern Norfolk (Moseley et al, 1977a) it has been shown that the first car is often used by the male head of household for a journey to work, and subsequent cars by other members of the household. The distribution of new car ownership between households which at present own no car, one car or more than one car is therefore crucial to any consideration of the implications of higher rates of car ownership for personal mobility. Seen in this light, car ownership expressed as a rate per household is a poor measure of the availability of cars to individual people. Table 2.7 shows car availability arranged in terms of different ownership categories.

Table 2.7
Car availability by household car ownership

Household owns:	0 cars %	1 car %	2 cars %	3 or more cars %
no licence	86	34	19	17
has licence, never has car	13	4	2	0
has licence, rarely has car	1	9	4	5
has licence, car nearly always	0	53	75	78
BASE	623	702	294	59

Source: Moseley et al (1977b)

The striking feature is that a substantial proportion of adults in car owning households are not able to drive and are therefore dependent upon being driven for priority trips such as those for medical purposes. In one car households (which are by far the most common) one third of the adult members do not have a driving licence, and this proportion is only reduced to 19% and 17% for two and three car households. As might be expected, the proportion of individuals who were recorded as having a car available for use nearly all of the time rises with increasing car ownership up to two cars, and remains steady

thereafter.   This "ceiling" effect is partially explained when we
consider the same figures disaggregated by sex (Table 2.8).

Table 2.8
Car availability by household car ownership and sex

Household owns:	0 cars		1 car		2 cars		3 or more cars	
	%M	%F	%M	%F	%M	%F	%M	%F
No licence	77	93	13	55	5	53	7	28
never has car	22	6	4	3	1	3	0	0
rarely has car	1	1	7	12	2	6	3	7
car nearly always	0	0	76	30	92	58	90	65
BASE	122	158	351	351	153	141	30	29

Source: Moseley et al (1977b)

It would seem that men tend to make most use of the first car,
although nearly a third of the women in this group were recorded as
having the use of a car for early all of the time.   In two car households this figure rises to nearly two thirds, but thereafter remains
constant with increasing car ownership, reflecting the high proportion
of women without a driving licence and the number of households in
which the second car (or subsequent cars) is used solely by a son or
daughter, or other member of the household.   Although it is the
acquisition of the second car which appears to affect the use a women
is able to make of a household car, a quarter of the women in households with two or more cars did not have a licence.

Of the sample interviewed in rural Norfolk in 1975, only 22% of men
did not have a driving licence, while 58% of women did not.   These
figures can be compared with similar figures from the National Travel
Survey conducted two years' earlier, which found 33% of men and 75%
of women without a licence (Department of the Environment, 1976a).
The lesser mobility of women compared with men does not, however,
obtain equally across all income groups.   Women in households with
higher incomes are much more likely to have a driving licence and to
have access to a car than women in low income households, when the
number of cars owned is held constant.   Table 2.9 illustrates this
phenomenon and shows that men's car use is not associated with income
in the same way.

The association between female car availability and age is also
worth attention.   Table 2.10 shows that for both men and women the
percentage without a licence increases with age, with the exception of
the youngest adult age group.   The lower rate of licence holding among
women is partly a result of historical influences, and we may expect
more women to be able to drive as the present population ages.

Table 2.9
Car availability for persons aged 17-61 by household income, sex and car ownership

Income	Household owns:	1 car			2 or more cars		
		No.	NL	CA	No.	NL	CA
Males							
under £2,000		63	7	85	7	0	100
£2,000- £4,000		96	7	71	49	2	95
more than £4,000		26	7	73	46	2	91
Females							
under £2,000		70	62	29	8	50	50
£2,000- £4,000		108	44	32	51	29	62
more than £4,000		25	32	40	44	15	65

No. = Number in cell
NL = percentage without a driving licence
CA = percentage with a car nearly always

Source: Moseley et al (1977b)

Table 2.10
Car availability (percentage without licence by age and sex)

Age	Male SWD	Male Married	Female SWD	Female Married
17-25	26	14	54	37
26-45	39	7	48	37
45-60	31	8	63	5?
61-65	40	26	79	74
over 65	64	41	89	88
All	38	17	71	53
BASE	174	482	192	487

SWD = Single, widowed and divorced

Source: Moseley et al (1977b)

It is noticeable that both males and females over the age of 61 have low rates of licence holding. The National Travel Survey found that 68% of retired men and 94% of retired females did not have a driving licence. In the Norfolk surveys 65% of elderly households did not have a car. The elderly, then, have much lower rates of licence holding and car ownership than the rest of the population. Other factors, such as their social and physical characteristics compound the problem arising from their low car availability. In the Norfolk

23

surveys one quarter of those over 61 years reported having serious difficulty in moving about (Moseley et al, 1977a). In Hillman's survey of pensioners, 32% said that they had some personal difficulty in getting about due to their physical condition (Hillman, 1976). This lack of physical mobility reduces the ability of the elderly to retain the use of a car, and furthermore makes the use of public transport more difficult.

The preceding analysis is based upon the assumption that the car availability category recorded for each respondent applied at all times. It is likely that in reality the use that each member of the household can make of the car(s) owned by that household will vary throughout the day (and by day of the week), and will also vary according to the importance attached to the trip. We may expect, for example, that women in one car households will be able to make more use of the household car in the evenings, when it is not being used by the man for a journey to work, and that medical trips will be considered as a relatively high priority trip purpose which will be reflected in a greater use of the household car. The Norfolk survey contained no information on the variation in car availability with time of day, but did include a study of trips to obtain medical treatment (all trips to doctors, dentists and other places of medical treatment were so defined). Although these trips are not directly relevant to the community hospital issue, they do shed some light on the way in which people with differing mobility characteristics make relatively high priority trips.

Table 2.11 shows the mode of transport used on medical trips for those without a licence and those with a car available for nearly all the time. For those with a car available, 91% of all trips are made by car and most of these trips are made as the driver. Only 21% of the car drivers were accompanied by another passenger. Those without a licence travel more on foot and by public transport than those with ready access to a car, but, even so, 64% of all trips by non-licence holders are made by car, a fairly large number being made as a passenger in a car not owned by the household. An informal "social car service" is evidently just as important as public transport in these communities.

Table 2.11
Mode used for medical trips by car availability of individual

	no licence %	car nearly always %
Walk/cycle	14	5
Driving household car	3	80
Passenger in household car	48	10
Other car passenger	13	1
Public transport	16	1
Other	6	4
BASE	223	164

Source: Moseley et al (1977b)

Accessibility of centres by car

For the majority of hospital out-patients and visitors to in-patients
who travel by car, which are the most convenient hospital locations
within the Health District? A good indicator of convenience and
assessibility is the time taken on the journey, and the time taken by
car is to a large extent predictable from the distance travelled.

Figure 2.3 is based on a survey of the journeys of out-patients in the
King's Lynn District (to be described in Chapter 4) and shows the trip
times expected to different centres from different places. The iso-
chrones (lines of equal time) are averages and do not take into account
the fact that progress on some roads may be faster and on others,
correspondingly slower. They serve to illustrate, however, the point
that virtually the whole health district is well within a 30 minute car
journey (including parking, etc.) of at least one of the following
centres: King's Lynn, Wisbech, Downham Market, Swaffham, Fakenham and
Hunstanton. Most of the district (with the exception of the eastern
and southern margins) is within a total time of 40 minutes from King's
Lynn itself. For the people in the eastern and southern margins the
journey time to King's Lynn will most likely be improved when their
destination in King's Lynn becomes a clinic at the new district general
hospital, which will have parking space at hand and which may be
approached by avoiding the town centre and its traffic.

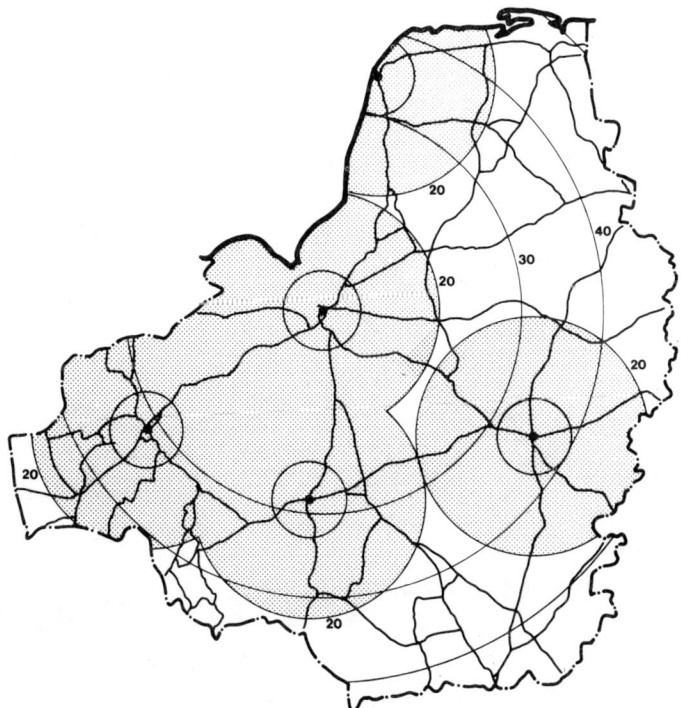

Figure 2.3   Average journey times by car

PUBLIC TRANSPORT

Present rail and bus services

The principal operators of public transport in the King's Lynn Health
District are Eastern Counties Omnibus Company (ECOC) and British Rail.
The Lincolnshire Road Car Company operates a route between Spalding and
King's Lynn.   ECOC and the Lincolnshire Road Car Company are not of
course the only stage carriage operators in the district.   There are
at least three private coach operators.   Small operators such as these
form an important element in the public transport provision in many
areas, and are easily overlooked.   Figure 2.4 shows the frequencies of
buses operated on a stage carriage basis throughout the year and the
passenger rail network in the area.   The bus network appears to be
dense, most settlements having a service of one kind or another but
many routes are operated at low frequencies, some being weekly or
twice weekly "market day" services.   It is unlikely that such services
can provide reasonable access to hospitals.

In order to classify parts of the district according to the level of
public transport enjoyed, bus timetables were scrutinised to establish
the number of buses passing through each parish regardless of destination.   Parishes were then grouped into those without any service,
those with at least one bus on at least one weekday, those with a service on five weekdays but less than 15 buses per day and those with more
than 15 buses per day (regardless of direction) for five days a week.

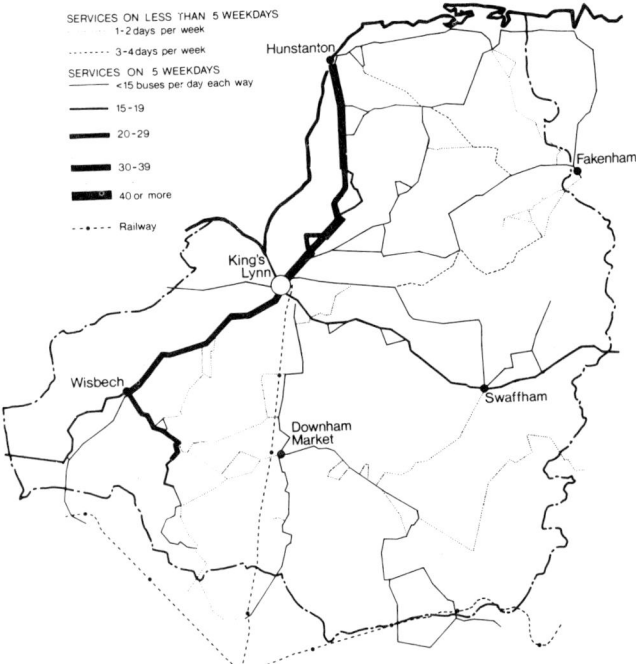

Figure 2.4   Public transport

Private bus operators were included, but rail services were not.
Parishes were chosen as the basic unit simply for convenience: if a
bus route passed through any part of a parish, it was considered to
serve the population of the parish. This is an over-simplification,
of course, but any other assumption would have been more difficult to
apply and would not necessarily have markedly improved the accuracy of
the analysis.   In most cases the parish boundaries are related to
settlement patterns and a bus route entering a parish almost always
passes through its main settlements.

Figure 2.4 shows that there are three main routes with more than 15
buses per day.   These routes link King's Lynn with Hunstanton, Wisbech
(and ultimately Peterborough) and Swaffham (on the way to Norwich).
The main settlements are served on a regular basis, but many areas have
a relatively poor service.   Table 2.12 shows the estimated population
with access to different levels of public transport.

Table 2.12
Estimated population with different levels of public transport

Bus service	Population served	
	numbers	% of district
on 5 days (15 buses per day or more)	90,592	58
on 5 days (less than 15 buses per day)	36,816	23
on 1 to 4 days per week	11,802	7
no service	18,101	12
TOTAL	157,311	100

In considering the quality of public transport account must be taken
not only of the frequency of buses passing through or near a particular
settlement, but also the cost, the purpose of the journey and its
destination, and the type of person who may wish to make trips.   A
market day service is unlikely to provide an adequate level of access
to out-patient clinics for example, as these services are only available
on certain days and may not arrive and depart at suitable times for a
morning or afternoon clinic appointment.   It is necessary, therefore,
to consider access to hospital by public transport in relation to the
timing of out-patient clinics and visiting sessions, as these are the
constraints within which a journey must be made.   There are also other
factors which contribute to the quality of transport, but which are not
in themselves absolute constraints.   Such things are the length of
time spent waiting for connections or the distance an individual must
walk to the bus stop, the time taken on the journey and its cost.
Of course, some of these factors affect some individuals to a greater
extent than the majority of people.   The elderly, those with physical
disability, women accompanied by children and other groups who have a
high dependence upon public transport have particular problems in
making use of buses.   The old and handicapped (often the same people)
may suffer when buses are unreliable and long waits in unsheltered
conditions must be endured.   Getting on and off the bus can have its
problems and a study undertaken by British Leyland on behalf of the

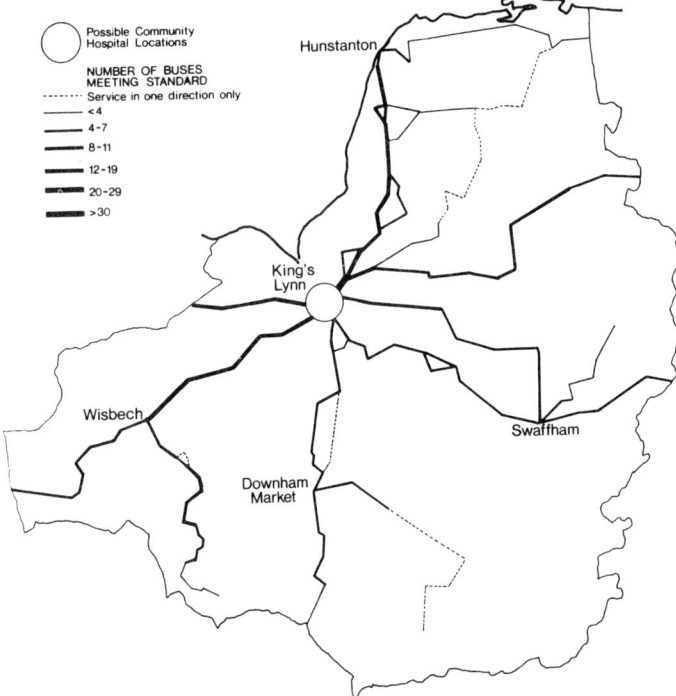

Figure 2.5   Bus service standards to King's Lynn

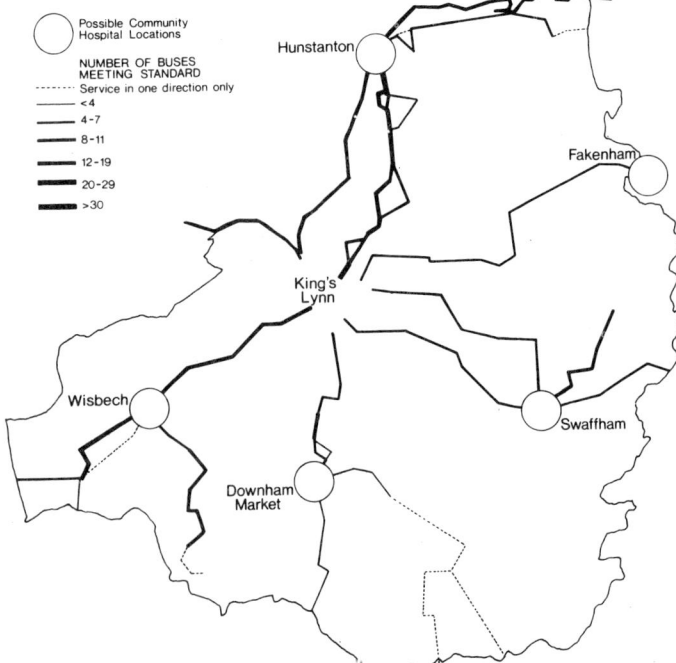

Figure 2.6   Bus service standards to other towns

Transport and Road Research Laboratory estimated that about four million people in the country (of which two million are over 65) could not manage a step height of seventeen inches, the legal limit (Brooks et al, 1974). Positioning of handrails and bells, visibility of destination signs, design of bus seating and the difficulties caused by one man operation make buses difficult (and possibly dangerous) for many elderly or handicapped people. Hillman (1976) found that elderly people in rural areas considered that unreliability, infrequency, waiting and effort (which was mainly associated with getting on and off the bus) were major problems associated with the use of buses, and were more of a deterrent to them than cost.

Figures 2.5 and 2.6 attempt to show how access by public transport varies when simple standards are applied. Figure 2.5 shows the situation for services to King's Lynn, and Figure 2.6 covers services to Hunstanton, Fakenham, Swaffham, Downham Market and Wisbech. The maps show the number of buses allowing an inward journey departing after 08.00 and arriving at the destination before 15.00 and an outward journey departing after 12.00 and arriving before 19.00. Where only one leg of the journey is possible within these times it is shown as a broken line. Connecting services via King's Lynn are not shown on Figure 2.6. Within each town the distances from the alighting point to the hospital (or ultimate destination) were ignored; but very few of the buses serving Downham Market, for example, pass near the hospital at the moment. Similarly, with current bus routes and frequencies, the new district general hospital site in King's Lynn will be less accessible than the existing hospitals. Most bus users will need to change buses in King's Lynn in order to reach the new peripheral location.

In terms of the places served, King's Lynn has a much higher level of service than any of the other centres. The other towns have bus links to fewer places, although all can be reached from King's Lynn itself. The pattern of services shown in the maps demonstrates a common feature of rural public transport; the high frequency routes are essentially inter-urban, and are not arranged primarily to serve the rural areas or to feed the small market towns from their surrounding hinterlands. Market towns may have relatively good services, but these usually arise because they lie on a route linking the main towns of the wider area. Swaffham, for example, is on the King's Lynn-Norwich route, and has a service to both these centres. It does not have a daily service to any of the villages to the south.

Figure 2.7 shows the extent of public transport services to five possible community hospital locations. All parishes with a return service with more than 15 buses per day in either direction for five days a week are considered to have access to the appropriate hospital location. Where a parish has access to more than one hospital location (and in all cases King's Lynn is one of these) an arbitrary boundary (shown as a broken line) is indicated approximately halfway between the centres. The resulting pattern is far from ideal, many areas having no service of the required standard to one of the possible hospital sites, and catchments reflecting the linear nature of the bus services. The pattern of public transport accessibility shown, incomplete as it is, certainly errs on the generous side, not only because the timing of certain services might be inconvenient but because

many individuals will have difficulty in making use of the public
transport that appears to be available to them.

As a group, the elderly depend more on public transport and, para-
doxically, are less able to use it than the general population.   The
distribution of elderly people in the district is therefore of some
interest.   Figure 2.8 shows the parishes with high and low proportions
of elderly in the population.   The information was taken from the 1971
census small area statistics, and "elderly" in this context was defined
as men over the age of 65 and women over the age of 60.   The map shows
that a high proportion of the population in parishes in the north of
the district is elderly.   Because these parishes contain fewer people
than most parishes elsewhere in the district, the elderly people in
the north are only a small proportion of all elderly in the district.
Nevertheless, the northern area is expected to have particular problems.
The high proportion of elderly persons may represent an even greater
proportion of households than of people and the fact that car ownership and income levels may be lower than elsewhere reduces the ability
of the community to seek its own solutions to accessibility problems.
In areas where retirement migration is an important factor the separa-
tion of the elderly from other members of their families may compound
these problems.   Another disadvantaged group consists of people with
low socio-economic status, for, as was seen earlier, these people are
less likely to own cars than the general population and consequently
are more dependent upon public transport.   Figure 2.9 shows the location of parishes with high and low proportions of semi- and unskilled
manual workers (census socio-economic groups 10, 11 and 15, from the
1971 census small area statistics: 10% sample).

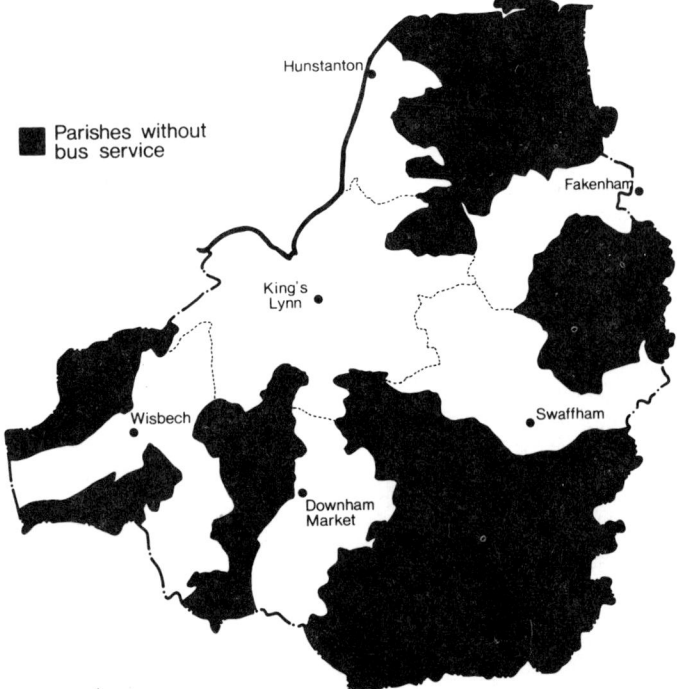

Figure 2.7   Access to potential community hospital locations

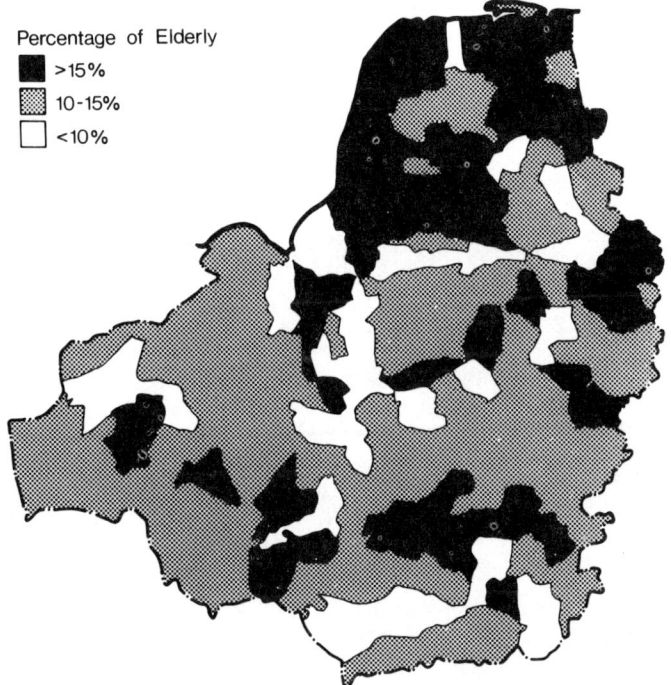

Figure 2.8   Distribution of elderly people

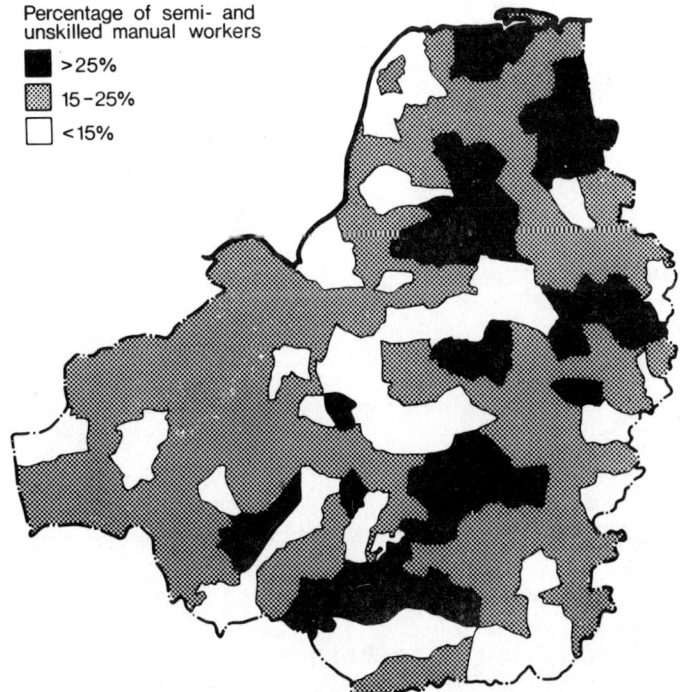

Figure 2.9   Distribution of semi- and unskilled manual workers

Unlike the distribution of elderly people, Figure 2.9 does not indicate a cluster in the northern area.   There is no obvious pattern in the parishes with a high proportion of semi- and unskilled manual workers, except that visual comparison with the maps of public transport suggests that perhaps these parishes tend to be poorly served by buses.

A means of comparing the distribution of various groups with public transport provision is given in Table 2.13, which is based upon the classification of parishes into four different categories of public transport quality.   This table supports the suggestion that the lower socio-economic groups form a greater proportion of the population in areas with poor bus services.   The areas with poor bus services do have higher rates of car ownership, but it is not possible to tell whether this higher car ownerhip is concentrated within the higher socio-economic groups or whether it is what might be termed "forced" car ownership amongst poorer people.   Table 2.13 also shows that 19% of the district's elderly population live in parishes which do not have a five days a week bus service.   A slightly lower percentage (17%) of the retired migrants who moved into the district in the period 1966-1971 moved to these very badly served parishes.   It will be recalled from Table 2.12 that altogether such parishes (which must be considered almost totally inaccessible by public transport to hospital facilities) account for 19% of the district's population.   Of the remainder, another 23% live in parishes with less than 15 buses a day, and 58% enjoy the benefits of more than 15 buses a day.

Table 2.13

Population characteristics for zones with different levels of public transport

Population sub-group	5 day (15+ buses)	5 day (<15 buses)	1 - 4 day	no service
Semi- and unskilled manual workers as % of zone population*	15	18	21	17
Households owning at least 1 car as % of zone households	60	68	66	70
Households owning at least 2 cars as % of zone households	10	15	15	13
Elderly population as % of zone population	18	18	20	14
Elderly population as % of district elderly populatior.	59	22	7	12
1966-71 elderly migrants as % of district elderly migrants*	66	16	6	11

* 10% sample census   Source: 1971 census

While the frequency, reliability and convenience of rural bus services are arguably more important factors for most people than their cost (especially in the context of high priority medical trips), cost may be expected to assume greater significance for patients who need to make regular trips to an out-patient clinic and for visitors to long-stay hospital in-patients. Figures 2.10 and 2.11 illustrate the current (February 1978) single fares operating from the six towns in or near the district. As can be seen from the maps, single fares of 50 pence or greater (implying a return cost exceeding £1) are not uncommon for the journey to King's Lynn. For people who travel to their nearest market town, single fares range from 20 to 40 pence, except for the south-eastern part of the district, where single fares to Wisbech exceed 50 pence. Bearing in mind that out-patients and visitors to hospitals often do not travel alone but are accompanied, it seems likely that the cost of public transport might be a considerable burden for some people. Eastern Counties Omnibus Company does sell a ten trip ticket, valid for three months, which enables passengers to obtain a 10% discount if regular trips to a hospital are necessary, but even with this discount costs remain high.

Future levels of public transport

Is there a way to forecast the future of conventional stage carriage operations which will allow us to estimate access to hospitals at some future date? Unfortunately there is not, although we may look at past trends, government attitudes to subsidy and some new developments in rural public transport to provide a framework for discussion of the topic.

Between 1954 and 1974 the bus mileage operated per annum by ECOC in the Norwich area fell by 19.4% in the city of Norwich, and by 26.5% in the county. Table 2.14 shows national figures for stage carriage operations which indicate that there has been a decline of nearly 22% in vehicle mileages during the last half of the same period.

Table 2.14
Vehicle kms covered by stage carriage operations 1964-1975

			(millions kms)		
1964	3,053	1968	2,775	1972	2,459
1965	2,971	1969	2,691	1973	2,411
1966	2,911	1970	2,567	1974	2,360
1967	2,848	1971	2,550	1975	2,396

Source: Department of Transport (1977)

It would be unreasonable to expect a reversal of the trends identified above in the foreseeable future. The decline in rural services in Norfolk has been a very gradual one, but from an already low base. In areas where the network of services is not dense and services are relatively infrequent even a small reduction may have far-reaching effects. However, for the short term at least, rural bus services are unlikely to disappear, but will continue to be supported by Government. The Central Government's attitude towards rural public

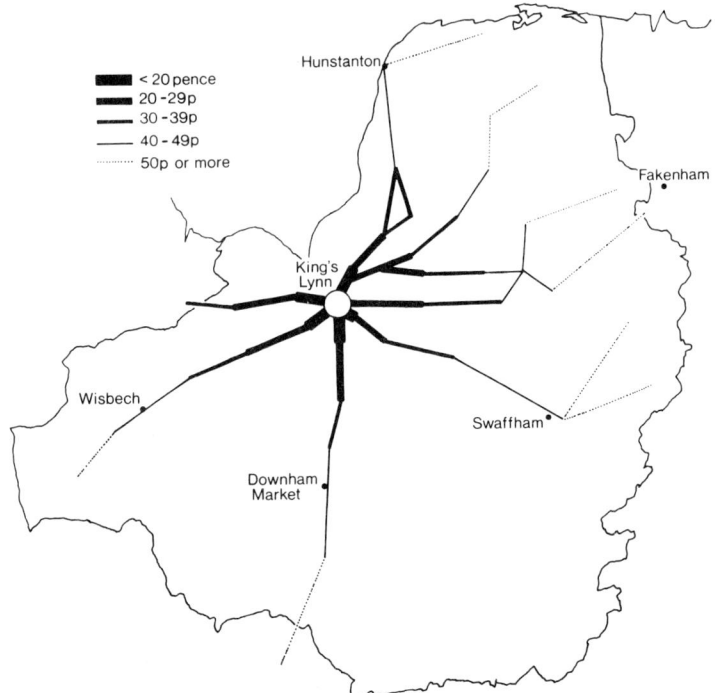

Figure 2.10   Single bus fares to King's Lynn

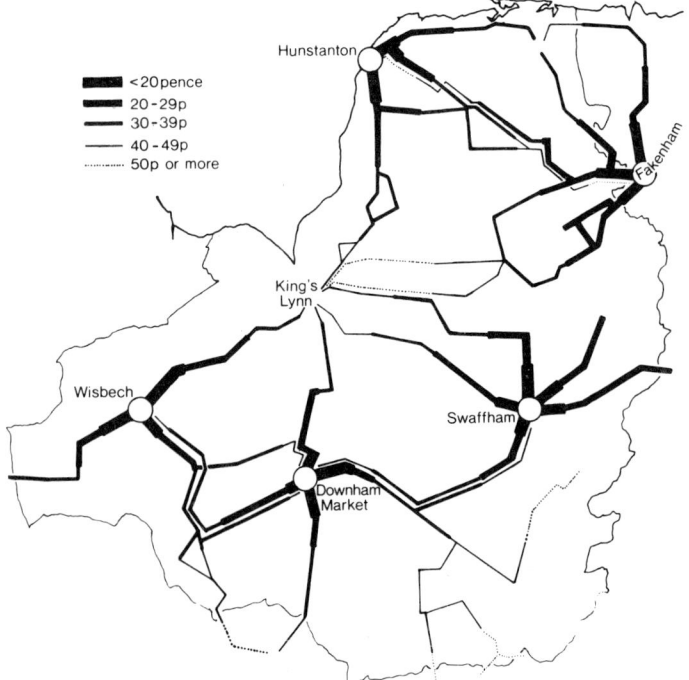

Figure 2.11   Single bus fares to other towns

transport subsidy has been recently restated in the White Paper on
Transport Policy (Cmnd. 6836, 1977) which reversed the proposal contained in the consultation document on transport policy published earlier
(Department of the Environment, 1976b) to reduce the provision for
financial support to local bus services by roughly half by the end of
the decade.   Instead, the provision for bus support will remain at the
current level of £150 million for the next few years.   In the rural
areas the White Paper proposes an increase in the annual provision for
rural services of about £15 million.

Local authorities are empowered under section 203 of the Local
Government Act, 1972, to make grants to subsidise certain bus routes,
and some of them operate concessionary fare schemes for the elderly
and the disabled.   They are also involved in transport planning
through their interest in the statutory town and country planning process
(primarily through the preparation of Structure Plans, Local Plans and
Transport Policies and Programmes) and through the work of the Transport
Co-ordinating Officer.

It is in the area of making the most of existing services rather
than attempting to regain the service levels of twenty years ago that
improvements may realistically be expected.   As far as conventional
stage carriage operations are concerned, what appears to be required
is closer liaison between the local authority, health authorities,
public transport companies and other interested bodies to allow discussion about possible overlapping services and adjustments to existing
services.   Possibly buses could be timed and routed to suit hospital
appointment systems, or appointments could be arranged to suit bus
services.   More publicity might be given to timetables and special
timetables for hospital services which include all operators might be
produced.   In this connection, we understand that Cambridgeshire
County Council and ECOC are currently working on timetable leaflets
which make clearer the routes and times of buses serving hospitals in
the Peterborough area.

There have been a number of innovations in rural public transport in
recent years and the National Bus Company, the Post Office and the
Transport and Road Research Laboratory are at present running experimental schemes.   Three community minibus experiments (in Norfolk, Wales
and East Suffolk) have been acknowledged as successful and the National
Bus Company is promoting the idea in suitable areas.   These schemes
rely on community operation of a minibus for all travel purposes.
The National Bus Company helps with licensing, insurance, vehicle
maintenance, publicity and driver training, and the county council
provide financial support and policy guidance.   By 1987 the company
estimates that about a thousand such schemes could be in operation.

Other minibus schemes involve vehicles owned by voluntary bodies or
hired to them.   These may be for particular purposes, such as elderly
persons' luncheon clubs, outings clubs, general practitioner surgery
visits, etc., or may be for a variety of trip purposes.   Vehicles
owned by one group may be hired to another to maximise use and revenue.
The legal situation, however, is very complex, especially with respect
to some of the quasi-public transport operations.

A third general area of improvement for "public" transport in rural areas is the development of voluntary transport using private cars. Many locally organised car pools and social car schemes already exist, and they are capable of satisfying both particular needs and general transport requirements. An essential pre-requisite is the local organiser, through whom all requests are channelled and drivers recruited. Groups such as WRVS might administer such schemes and local authority aid in the form of grants is a possibility. Local hospital car services run by voluntary bodies and partly funded by hospital leagues of friends could well capitalise upon the goodwill shown by the community towards local hospitals.

Proposed changes in legislation to facilitate community minibus schemes and remove legal obstacles to car sharing are expected to increase the attractiveness of these alternative means of transport. It must be stressed, however, that all unconventional public transport schemes rely to a large extent upon mobilising community resources and the time, experience and abilities of a few individuals. None are universally applicable, and few will provide a level of service comparable to that provided by a reasonably frequent conventional bus service. We can expect more of such schemes in the more remote rural areas (with possibly a concomitant decline in conventional operations). The new services could be more flexible than normal stage carriage operations and would have the potential to offer adequate access to local hospitals, provided that there is an enthusiastic and co-ordinated response from transport and hospital organisers.

NATIONAL HEALTH SERVICE TRANSPORT

In the public imagination the main role of ambulances is in accident and emergency work, but this is far from being true. In terms of the number of patients involved, the primary function of ambulances is to fill in the gaps of the private and public transport systems for routine and non-urgent trips to hospital. As Norman has described it:

"The bulk of the ambulance service's work is in transporting elderly people to hospital for out-patients' appointments and treatment. This was made clear as early as 1962/3 by the Hospital Organisation and Methods Service report which estimated approximately 83% of the 18.5 million patient journeys made by ambulance were for out-patients' appointments and only 6% for accident and emergency. Between 60% and 70% of the out-patient journeys were for physiotherapy, orthopaedic and fractures. The figures were not broken down for age but the report concludes that the vast majority of these patients were elderly. Numbers have increased since then, but the general picture has not changed." (Norman, 1977, p.65).

The gradual decline in rural public transport since 1963 has meant that ambulances and the hospital car service (especially the latter) have to some extent become substitutes for the bus. However, indications that rural dwellers make less trips to clinics than townspeople may be evidence that these forms of National Health Service transport are able only partially to fill the gaps in rural transport

Table 2.15
Vehicle mileage

Year	Ambulance	Car Service
1975	1,343,398	2,334,878
1976	1,399,014	2,817,954
1977 (estimate)	1,577,452	2,969,218

Table 2.16
Patients conveyed

	Ambulance			Car Service		
	1975	1976	1977*	1975	1976	1977*
Emergency	13,166	16,120	19,750	-	-	-
All other	114,151	116,019	118,950	215,254	226,393	235,644

* Estimate

Table 2.17
Vehicles miles per patient

Year	Ambulance	Car Service
1975	10.55	10.85
1976	10.59	12.45
1977 (estimate)	11.37	12.60

Table 2.18
Cost per vehicle mile

Year	Ambulance	Car Service
1975	£0.61	£0.11
1976	£0.95	£0.12
1977 (estimate)	£0.93	£0.14

services.

In England there are considerable variations in ambulance and car
service use between area health authorities. The average number of
miles travelled per patient tends to be considerably higher in the
rural areas. For example, in 1976 the figure for all health service
modes for Norfolk was 11.6 miles whereas some typical values for urban
areas are Greater London (4.8 miles per patient), Merseyside (4.5 miles
per patient) and the West Midlands (5.3 miles per patient). These
figures were taken from Form SBH 195, supplied by the Statistics
Division of DHSS.

The King's Lynn Health District is served primarily by Norfolk Area
ambulance stations in King's Lynn, Swaffham, Fakenham, Downham Market
and Hunstanton, and the Cambridge Area station in Wisbech. As ambulance service statistics are collected on an Area basis, we shall
concentrate on those applicable to Norfolk as a whole. The information
contained in Tables 2.15 to 2.19 has been provided by the Norfolk Area
Ambulance Service.

As can be seen from Table 2.15, ambulance mileage in Norfolk has been
estimated as increasing by 16% in the last three years and the mileage
of the car service has similarly increased by about 27%. These increases
in mileage have not been proportionally matched by increases in the
number of non-emergency patients conveyed (the ambulance service had an
estimated 4% increase and the car service an estimated 9% increase in
patients). Consequently, the average number of vehicle miles per
patient has increased during the period for both modes of transport.
The reason for this phenomenon is not known, but it is possible that as
an ambulance service expands its operations the people in more remote
areas are offered a proportionately greater share of its use. Another
possibility is that ambulance and car occupancy rates have been decreasing. In Table 2.17, vehicle miles per patient is calculated by dividing
total vehicle miles by total patient numbers. A more useful measure
of average number of miles per patient would need to incorporate information on the frequencies with which ambulances and hospital car
service vehicles carry different numbers of patients together.

Table 2.19
Cost per patient

Year	Ambulance	Car Service
1975	£6.46	£1.27
1976	£10.11	£1.53
1977 (estimate)	£10.54	£1.83

Table 2.19 shows that the cost per patient has risen over the last
three years by 63% for the ambulance service and 44% for the car
service. Since no allowance has been made for inflation, the slight
increase in ambulance costs in Tables 2.20 and 2.21 from 1976 to 1977
is misleading: what is shown amounts to a decrease in real cost terms.
The cost figures are based on an accounting practice which includes all

expenditure (whether investment or current) in the calculation of average costs per patient or per mile and they must therefore be treated with great caution. Furthermore, current expenditure includes costs which are incurred semi-independently of the number of patients conveyed or the number of miles travelled (for example, administrative costs, central office overheads, non-ambulance vehicle costs, etc.), and yet these costs are included in the costs per patient and the cost per mile for the ambulance service. They are not, however, included in the costs of the car service, whose administrative costs are account-ed for under the ambulance service. The result of this procedure is that the ambulance costs are serious over-estimates, which cannot be used to predict the likely increase in costs if, for example, the number of patients conveyed or the total mileage were to increase slightly.

It was originally hoped to cost the implications of the community hospital policy with respect to the movement of patients by the ambulance service, but it is unlikely that an attempt to do this would be useful without more detailed statistics on the marginal costs involved. We shall therefore devote our main attention not to the costs, but to the number of patient miles likely to be required of the ambulance and car services under different hospital arrangements. The ambulance service has critical importance in the community hospital policy, especially with regard to day care, in that it will act as a rationing mechanism. Those who can be transported to day care services are the ones who will benefit, whether or not they are the patients who are most in need.

SUMMARY

The King's Lynn Health District is a predominantly rural area. King's Lynn and Wisbech are the most important towns. Other than those the only urban settlements are the small market towns of Swaffham and Downham Market and the small holiday resort of Hunstanton. The population is growing slowly and this growth is expected to continue. However, there are marked variations within the area. In some of the remoter rural areas there is substantial out-migration and an age-ing population. Around King's Lynn there are rapidly growing commuter villages with a predominantly youthful population.

The main hospitals of the district are concentrated in King's Lynn and Wisbech, although there are currently some smaller hospitals else-where. The district is seriously under-provided with hospital facilities in a number of specialties, facilities for the elderly and the mentally ill being particularly lacking. The quality of some of the existing provision is also poor. However, the hospital services of the district will be radically changed by the opening of a new district general hospital in King's Lynn in 1980. Although this will provide new beds in many specialities it will also be very costly and financial limits will necessitate the closure of many existing hospital facilities. Therefore, the current proposals by the Area Health Authority envisage an increasing concentration of the hospital services of the district in the town of King's Lynn, while leaving open the possibility of developing community hospital units elsewhere.

There are a number of important features of the transport system of the district which affect the accessibility of hospitals to the population. About seven out of every ten households in the King's Lynn Health District own at least one car. Adult members of households which own a car do not have equal use of it, indeed one third of them are not able to drive, but trips to hospital have a high priority and are expected to attract a very high proportion of car trips from car owning households. Including the additional lifts given to non car owners in cars belonging to friends or relatives, car trips to out-patient clinics or to visit hospital patients are expected to account for more than 70% of hospital trips which are beyond walking distance. All the market towns in the King's Lynn District are conveniently accessible by car from their surrounding areas and the total journey time to a hospital in King's Lynn itself would rarely exceed 40 minutes. Accessibility in the King's Lynn District is not a serious problem for car users.

Even with a steady rise in car ownership, a large minority of the population will remain dependent upon public transport. Particularly the elderly, but also other groups such as the poor, single person households and lower-income women, have to rely on the bus service for transport outside the village. Examination of bus timetables has shown that the image of the rural bus connecting each market town with its surrounding rural catchment area is largely a myth. For the most part, rural bus services in the King's Lynn District link the places which happen to lie on the main routes between towns. Handicapped or frail people may not be able to use the bus, but even for those who are physically able there simply may be no service to use.

The extent of trip suppression caused by transport difficulties is not known, but part of the gap is filled by ambulances and the hospital car service. Present accounting practices make it difficult to compare the real costs involved, but it seems that the hospital car service is a mode of transport much more appropriate to this function than the ambulance service. Using skilled ambulance personnel and specialised vehicles to ferry people to and from out-patient departments is an expensive and inefficient use of resources.

In some respects the problems of access to hospitals cannot be separated from the rural transport problem in general; the movement of people to hospital is just one aspect of this, whether it is in a hospital car service vehicle, an ambulance, on a public bus or train, or in a private car. The agencies involved in providing public transport (in its widest sense) are numerous and functionally diverse. The include local private, municipal and National Bus Company stage carriage operators, the education and social services departments of local authorities, the ambulance service, the Post Office (through the operation of postbuses) and voluntary bodies. In some cases these bodies also make decisions which affect the location of facilities. The framework for better liaison exists and the different functions of these agencies should not obscure their common accessibility problems.

3 The feasibility and functions of rural community hospitals

Community hospitals are likely to be most successful where they are seen to be meeting important needs in an efficient manner. The extent to which the medical profession feels that they will be able to do this is therefore a very important issue. Not only will this influence their general attitude to the community hospital policy, but also it will have an important bearing on whether they are prepared to be actively involved in community hospitals. Such involvement will be absolutely vital for the success of community hospitals. They will have to rely on general practitioners to provide the day to day medical care of patients whilst consultants will have to be willing to release patients and to hold out-patient clinics in the community hospitals. Furthermore, for community hospitals to provide a high standard of care for their patients they will have to be able to attract high calibre nurses and other professional staff such as physiotherapists, occupational therapists and radiographers.

However, no matter how attractive community hospitals might appear to medical staff, if they are too costly they are unlikely to be successful. An important question, therefore, must be how the costs of caring for patients in a community hospital compare with the costs of caring for these patients in other ways, and how these costs vary with the size of the community hospital.

THE SIGNIFICANCE OF HEALTH SERVICE STAFF ATTITUDES

One of the major issues facing community hospital policy is whether doctors feel that these hospitals will provide a satisfactory level of care for their patients. In the community hospital circular it is argued that a considerable proportion of patients now in general hospitals either never needed or no longer need the full diagnostic and treatment facilities of these hospitals. The policy therefore implies that consultants should be prepared to release some of their patients to community hospitals. A major question must be to what extent are they prepared to do this? How does this vary by specialty? Does the proportion they would be prepared to release depend on whether they would maintain some control over the treatment of the patients in the community hospital? Clearly, if consultants are prepared only to release a small proportion of their patients the aim that community hospitals should ease the pressure on the district general hospitals will not be fully met.

However, the community hospital policy does not only imply a simple transfer of suitable patients from a district general hospital to a community hospital as many people who are not in hospital could be admitted. For example, patients with chronic disabilities might be admitted for short periods whilst their families, who normally look after them, are ill or on holiday. Therefore, another major issue is

41

whether there is currently an unmet need for hospital beds for certain groups of patients. Being in the front line of medical care, the general practitioner is in a very good position to judge whether such unmet needs exist. Furthermore, the extent to which community hospitals are seen as providing an improvement in the care that can be offered to such patients will influence the general practitioner's willingness to co-operate with the community hospital policy.

The views of the medical profession will also be important for the types of functions that a community hospital should perform. The original DHSS guidelines are fairly clear on what a community hospital should do and what it should not. In general it is proposed that they should provide medical and nursing care for those people who do not need the specialised facilities of the district general hospital but who cannot be satisfactorily cared for at home. Thus, they would provide up to half of the geriatric beds for a district, most of the beds for elderly patients with dementia and up to a fifth of medical and surgical beds mostly for general medical and preconvalescent patients. They would not be expected to provide accident and emergency facilities, only minor surgery would be considered appropriate and they would not normally be expected to have maternity delivery facilities. Many doctors are likely to have definite opinions on the appropriateness of this range of functions and the degree to which they agree with the DHSS guidelines will probably also influence their will-ingness to co-operate in community hospital developments.

In addition to their general views on the policy, another extremely important question is whether doctors would actually be prepared to work in community hospitals. The DHSS proposes that general practit-ioners would be responsible for the day to day medical care of patients in community hospitals. Therefore, the establishment of such hospitals will only be possible where there are sufficient GPs willing and able to provide the necessary care. Much will depend on the enthusiasm of GPs for this type of work, what distances they are prepared to travel and the conditions of service offered to them. The feasibility of holding out-patients clinics at community hospitals will likewise depend on the attitudes of consultants as to the appropriateness of such clinics for their specialty and on their willingness to hold them. Without the enthusiasm and the active involvement of many general practitioners and consultants community hospitals in the form envisaged will not be possible.

In addition to involving local GPs and consultants, community hospitals will also need to attract nurses and other trained staff such as physio-therapists, occupational therapists and radiographers. Are small hospitals attractive to these people? Will small, local hospitals with a high proportion of elderly patients, some of whom may be mentally infirm, be able to compete with district general hospitals for the staff which are available? Do the small market towns, which are expected to be the locations for community hospitals in many rural areas, have sufficient reserves of skilled staff? Perhaps these places contain such people who are not presently working but who would wish to work if there were the opportunity locally. If such reserves are not avail-able it might be possible to staff the community hospitals only by depleting the district hospitals to scarce staff. Answers to questions like these will be of great importance for the viability of community hospital policy.

THE QUESTIONNAIRE SURVEYS OF STAFF

In view of the importance that health service staff attitudes will have for community hospital policy an attempt has been made to assess such attitudes by conducting questionnaire surveys in the King's Lynn District. One survey was concerned with hospital doctors, another with general practitioners and the third with nurses and other profess- ional staff.

In July 1977 postal surveys of all hospital doctors and all general practitioners working in the King's Lynn District were carried out. Hospital doctors were sent a four page questionnaire (Appendix A), and general practitioners one of six pages (Appendix B). Both groups were also sent a five page extract from the DHSS circular (HSC(IS)75) on community hospitals. The accompanying letter explained that the circular was enclosed for interest: it was not necessary to read it before answering the questionnaire as a brief summary of the policy was included on the questionnaire form itself. A month after the original request all doctors who had not yet replied were sent another letter requesting their assistance, again with a copy of the question- naire form.

Completed forms were received from 69 of the hundred hospital doctors working in the district. The specialty and grade of each respondent were obtained not from the questionnaire form but from the Health District Office. The specialties represented in the replies are: anaesthetics, cardiology, chest diseases, cytology, dental surgery, dermatology, E.N.T., geriatric medicine, medicine, obstetrics and gynaecology, opthamology, orthopaedics, paediatrics, pathology, psy- chiatry, rheumetology, radiology, radiotherapy, surgery, thoracic surgery, and urology. More replies were received from consultants, both in terms of absolute numbers and in terms of the proportional response, than other grades of hospital doctor (Table 3.1). The response rate for consultants was 79% and for non-consultant doctors 58%.

Table 3.1
Grades of hospital doctor respondents

Grade	Number of Respondents	Number in the District
Consultant	38	48
Registrar	6	14
Senior House Officer	16	26
House Officer	2	5
Medical Assistant	2	3
Clinical Assistant	2	4

As Table 3.2 shows, the respondents varied in age from under 30 to over 60, with the most common age category in the middle (40-49) and a lesser mode in the under 30 category. Only six respondents were over 59 years old.

Table 3.2
Age of hospital doctors

Age	Number of respondents
Under 30	16
30-39	14
40-49	22
50-59	11
60 and over	6

Completed forms were received from 70 of the 85 general practitioners, a response rate of 82%. Most respondents worked in partnerships, many of which were fairly small (Table 3.3). They ranged in age from under 30 to over 60 (Table 3.4). Approximately half had been in their present practice for five or less years but most of the remainder had been there for eleven or more years. 61% had main surgery premises which were purpose-built. Personal NHS lists varied considerably in size, as Table 3.5 shows.

Table 3.3
Number of general practitioners in partnerships

Size of Partnership	Number of respondents
Not in partnership	2
Partnership of 3 or less	36
Partnership of 4 or more	32

Table 3.4
Age of general practitioners

Age	Number of respondents
Under 30	4
30-39	27
40-49	20
50-59	15
60 and over	4

Table 3.5
Personal NHS list size

List size	Number of respondents
0- 999	4
1,000-1,499	1
1,500-1,999	12
2,000-2,499	25
2,500-2,999	16
3,000-3,499	12
3,500+	0

As an indication of the pool of expertise among the respondents, a question was asked about higher qualifications. Higher qualifications were held by 42 of the 70 general practitioners who replied. Much the most common higher qualification represented was the Diploma of the Royal College of Obstetricians and Gynaecologists, which 39% held. Apart from membership of the Royal College of General Practitioners, no other higher qualification dominates. Of the GPs surveyed, 80% had held a post-registration hospital appointment, mostly at senior house officer level. By far the most hospital experience had been gained in obstetrics and gynaecology. Almost half the respondents had held post-registration appointments in this specialty. In second place was a group of specialties containing general medicine, general surgery, paediatrics and casualty. One fifth to one quarter of the sampled GPs had experience in each of these. Other specialties were much further behind. A notable example is geriatrics, in which only 6% of respondents had post-registration hospital experience. At the time of the survey fourteen GPs held a hospital appointment and of those nine held clinical assistantships.

Nurses, physiotherapists, occupational therapists and radiographers working in the King's Lynn Health District were also sent a questionnaire form (Appendix C). All physiotherapists, occupational therapists, radiographers and nursing staff of the rank nursing officer and above were included. A sample of one third of the remaining nurses, stratified by grade and hospital, was taken. No student nurses or students in the other occupational groups were included and staff working in maternity and psychiatric hospitals were excluded as community hospitals were considered unlikely to provide maternity and psychiatric services. Altogether, qualified staff in eight hospitals were involved. The hospitals were the West Norfolk and King's Lynn General Hospital, St. James' Hospital and Hardwick Hospital in King's Lynn, the North Cambridgeshire and Clarkson Hospitals in Wisbech, Stow Hall Hospital near Downham Market, the Swaffham Cottage Hospital and the Hunstanton Home of Recovery.

For nursing staff a response rate of 72% was obtained without a reminder. Table 3.6 gives the pattern of response by grade.

Table 3.6
Response by nursing staff

Grade	Number in sample	Number of Respondents
Divisional Nursing Officer	1	1
Senior Nursing Officer	3	1
Nursing Officer	13	11
Sister	26	23
Staff Nurse	41	23
S.E.N.	33	25
Total	117	84

A response rate of 72% was also achieved without a reminder for radiographers, physiotherapists and occupational therapists. Table 3.7 shows the pattern of response within each occupational group.

Table 3.7
Response by other occupational groups

Group	Number in sample	Number of Respondents
Radiography	13	11
Physiotherapy	20	12
Occupational therapy	10	8
Total	43	31

Ages were spread in the range 20-60, with a preponderance in the younger categories. 86% of respondents were women and 68% of respondents were married. A total of 40 (48%) of the nurses and 11 (35%) of the other groups were working part-time.

DOCTORS VIEWS ON COMMUNITY HOSPITALS

The views of general practitioners on the adequacy of existing hospital and other services

General practitioners were questioned about their views on the adequacy of aspects of the hospital service in the King's Lynn District. Of particular interest was whether there were certain groups of patients whose needs were not being properly met and whose position might be improved by the development of community hospitals in the area

Table 3.8

Views on adequacy of aspects of the hospital service in King's
Lynn district

	Adequate	Inadequate	Most Inadequate
Elderly acute admissions	57	6	5
Elderly chronic admissions	21	27	20
Admissions on social grounds	13	24	21
Information on patients in hospital	30	21	15
Speed of information after in-patient discharge	47	19	1
Information on out-patients	58	8	1

Table 3.8 shows that the majority of GPs thought that arrangements
for admitting elderly acute patients into hospital were generally
adequate. The same was true of information received following the
visit of patients to an out-patient clinic. A majority also thought
that the speed of information received from hospital following the
discharge of patients was adequate, although a sizeable minority
considered this to be inadequate. However, in respect of three
aspects of the hospital service a majority of the GPs thought that the
service was inadequate. These were the arrangements for admitting
elderly chronic patients into hospital, arrangements for hospital
admissions on social grounds and the information received about patients
whilst they are in hospital. Of these, it was the arrangements for
admitting patients on social grounds which was considered to be least
adequate. Thus the results of the survey suggest dissatisfaction
with certain aspects of the hospital service in the district.

This finding was confirmed when the GPs were asked whether there
were any types of patients they had particular difficulty in getting
admitted to hospital. 74% of GPs said they did experience such
difficulties and of these 69% suggested that geriatric and elderly
mentally infirm patients provided the greatest problems.

Whilst Table 3.8 presents the opinions of all GPs considered
together and is therefore an accurate reflection of views of the whole
sample, it is possible that different groups of GPs might show different responses. Of particular interest is whether the answers for
GPs practising in the towns differed from those for their rural
counterparts. To explore this issue, the sample was divided into
two groups. The first comprised those GPs practising in King's Lynn
or Wisbech: an urban group working in close proximity to the main
hospitals of the district. The second consisted of all the other GPs
surveyed and was therefore largely a rural group although it should be
noted that several practised in small market towns. These GPs are
geographically more remote from the main hospitals than are their
counterparts in the two main towns. Table 3.9 shows that this "rural"
groups was considerably more dissatisfied with the arrangements for
admitting elderly chronic patients. The relationship was statistically
significant at the 0.05 level. They were also significantly more

dissatisfied with the information received about their patients whilst they are in hospital (Table 3.10). "Rural" GPs therefore appear to be at a disadvantage when compared with their urban counterparts. The reasons for this are no doubt complicated but it does seem likely that in some way these are related to the relative isolation of the GPs working outside the main towns.

Table 3.9
Views on adequacy of arrangements for admitting elderly chronic patients into hospital

	Adequate	Inadequate	Most Inadequate
Urban GPs	12	9	3
Rural GPs	9	18	17

Table 3.10
Views on adequacy of information received about patients whilst they are in hospital

	Adequate	Inadequate	Most Inadequate
Urban GPs	18	4	2
Rural GPs	12	17	13

It is interesting to note that the aspects of the hospital service considered to be inadequate by the GPs are those likely to be improved by the development of community hospitals. These should make it easier for GPs to get elderly chronic patients admitted to hospital. Admissions on social grounds should be easier and GPs should be better informed about the condition of their patients whilst they are in hospital.

The survey also collected opinions on the adequacy of a number of services such as those provided by district nurses, physiotherapists, health visitors, chiropodists, social workers, home helps, Meals on Wheels and voluntary associations. Most GPs thought that the district nursing service was adequate (Table 3.11). The same was true in respect of health visitors, social workers, home helps, Meals on Wheels and voluntary associations although for each of these a sizeable minority of GPs expressed some dissatisfaction. However, both the physiotherapy and the chiropody services were considered inadequate by a majority of the doctors. Many GPs complained that they had no direct access to the services of a physiotherapists and this was mirrored in the low level of recent contact with this service. With chiropody the main problem mentioned was the length of time patients had to wait before treatment. Once again, this was reflected in the low level of recent contact with the service.

Table 3.11

Views on adequacy of a number of services in the King's Lynn district
and contact with these services during the last month

	Adequacy of service			Contact	
	Adequate	Inadequate	Most Inadequate	Yes	No
District Nurses	62	5	1	54	14
Physiotherapists	12	20	27	11	49
Health Visitors	53	10	3	45	21
Chiropodists	14	21	29	23	43
Social Workers	49	14	5	37	31
Home Helps	46	20	2	30	38
Meals on Wheels	48	16	2	17	49
Voluntary Associations	44	11	1	9	47

From these results it is possible to conclude that community hospitals
would perform a useful function in the study district if they improved
access by GPs to physiotherapy and chiropody services. There seems to
be a strong case for the development of these services at the local
scale.

Doctors' attitudes towards the community hospital policy

The attitudes of hospital doctors and general practitioners towards
the DHSS community hospital policy were gauged by giving a very brief
description of the policy on the questionnaire form and then presenting respondents with a list of statements with which they were
requested to indicate their level of agreement, using a five point
scale. All the statements were thought to be controversial and all
have a bearing on the policy. Most are paraphrases from the DHSS
circular, but three of them have no connection with the circular and
were included because they express other relevant issues (statements
3, 8 and 9). All the statements were related to the policy in a
positive way, that is to say, agreement with the statements indicate
agreement with the spirit of the policy and disagreement with one
implies disagreement with the other. The results for the two groups
of doctors are presented in Tables 3.12 and 3.13 in which the statements have been arranged so that the statement which is agreed with
most is at the top of the list and the statement which is agreed with
least is at the bottom. The index used to produce this ranking is
simply the number of responses in the "agree" and "strongly agree"
categories divided by the number of the "disagree" and "strongly
disagree" categories.

The most striking feature of the results is the high level of
agreement with the statements among the doctors sampled. Usually
the number of doctors in agreement with a statement exceeds the number
in disagreement by several times. In no case is the reverse true,
although one statement prompted a small majority of disagreements.
The responses in the "neither agree nor disagree" category are usually
not numerous and only for statement 10 do they exceed a third of all

responses, indicating perhaps that a large number of doctors felt this particular issue was too complex for simple overall agreement or disagreement.

The statements appear to divide themselves into three groups: those with which there was almost unanimous agreement, those in which there was a clear majority view and those which were more controversial.

Three of the statements prompted near unanimous agreement from both hospital doctors and general practitioners. The desirability of short-term admissions for elderly patients, the relative informality and relaxed atmosphere of small local hospitals and the desirability of hospital patients being able to keep in contact with relatives and friends are not contentious issues. Although nobody disagreed with the principle of short-term admissions for elderly patients, the comments given showed that several doctors were doubtful of its practicability - the problem is one of finding alternative accommodation. The quantity and quality of medical and nursing staff, it was pointed out, are other variables which affect the atmosphere of a hospital as well as size. Agreement with the idea that large hospital size adversely affects atmosphere does not, of course, identify the size at which the effect occurs. Even a general hospital, it was said, can still be "small" and "local". Few doctors denied that patients derive benefit from care near their homes so visiting is facilitated, but many explained that this benefit must be weighed against other benefits characteristic of larger and more distant hospitals.

The statement that consultants should hold out-patient clinics at small local hospitals also received unanimous support from the GPs. However, it is interesting to note that some hospital doctors, although only a minority, disagreed with this suggestion. Such clinics are clearly only suitable for certain specialties and, even in appropriate specialties, more consultant travelling time may mean fewer clinic attendances. We shall return to this question in more detail later and it will be shown that for their own specialty the ratio of doctors in favour of decentralised clinics is only 3:2. There seems therefore to be more enthusiasm for this proposal amongst GPs than amongst the hospital doctors who, as a group, would be responsible for providing the clinics.

There follows a series of statements which were agreed with by a majority, although not an overwhelming majority. There was widespread agreement that small local hospitals should not deal with more serious accident and emergency cases than a GP would in his surgery. A small minority of doctors commented that accident and emergency units must be both well equipped and local, but most respondents grasped the nettle and chose "well equipped" rather than "local" facilities. The statement that GPs should provide day to day medical treatment in small local hospitals was agreed by a ratio of more than 4:1. Indeed, more people declared themselves neutral (by marking the "neither" category) than disagreed with the statement. A number of respondents queried whether GPs have the time to provide the necessary commitment to this role. There were also several comments from GPs that their agreement with the statement was dependent on their being adequately financially rewarded for the job. Five hospital doctors volunteered

50

the view that even if a hospital is serviced largely by GPs, they should not be the patients' own GPs as the hospital work required full-time, specialty-oriented doctors. This is, of course, the opposite view to that which inspired the Wallingford experiment. Unfortunately the wording of the statement makes it impossible to claim that the 43 people who agreed with it also disagree with the idea of specialist "hospital GPs", but we think it is reasonable to assume that most respondents would consider that doctors described as "GPs" would serve a list of patients in domestic general practice.

On whether district nurses should also nurse patients in small local hospitals, the concensus was again strongly affirmative, which we consider a surprising result because, as far as we know, it is very rare for district nurses to look after patients in hospital as part of their duties. Of course, as with all these statements, doctors were asked to react to a rather abstract idea without being reminded of issues that would affect its practicability. Several doctors commented that district nurses already have too much work to do in the district and others were of the opinion that district nurses need not provide the main nursing care in small hospitals but should stay in touch by being based at the hospital or by helping occasionally. It is not part of the DHSS community hospital policy, but with a ratio of 3:1 hospital doctors in favour, the idea of involving district nurses in hospital work (or hospital nurses in district work) appears to merit some attention.

The last statement in the category of those which were agreed with by a clear majority is that the fear of hospitals felt by some elderly patients is often strong enough to impair the beneficial effects of hospital care. The policy implications appear to be either to make hospitals more like home or to treat susceptible patients at home as far as possible. Of those who disagreed with the statement, the strongest view was from a doctor who commented that in his experience only one in four hundred patients has any fear of hospital treatment. Fear of treatment is different from fear of hospital, perhaps, and it is not known to what extent these two reactions are confused in the attitudes reported here.

Next, there are four statements which seem to be rather more controversial. One of these concerns the extent to which surgical procedures should be carried out in small local hospitals. A substantial majority of hospital doctors agreed with the view that surgery in a community hospital should not extent beyond that which a GP would expect to perform in his own practice premises. Amongst GPs the issue was considerably more controversial. Opinion was fairly evenly balanced although with a small majority in agreement with the statement. Amongst those opposing the statement there were several comments that some GPs are sufficiently skilled and where the necessary facilities are provided they could usefully perform simple cold surgery and minor emergency work. In this context it should be noted that several of the GPs had post-registration hospital experience in surgery, although only one member of the sample had a higher qualification in surgery (primary FRCS).

51

Table 3.12
Hospital doctor's attitudes to issues (in order of agreement)

Statement	Strongly Agree	Agree	Neither	Disagree	Strongly Disagree	No reply
(8) Greater efforts should be made to admit elderly patients to hospital for short rather than long stays	23	32	6	0	0	8
(1) Small local hospitals seem less formal and forbidding to patients than larger hospitals	16	41	7	2	0	3
(2) Patients derive benefit from care in hospitals near their homes where they can easily be visited and maintain their links with the community	22	35	3	4	0	5
(11) No emergency or accident cases should be treated in a small local hospital other than those which would normally be dealt with in a GP's surgery	24	28	4	7	5	1
(4) Day to day medical care both of in-patients and day patients in small local hospitals should be provided by GPs	18	25	14	5	5	2
(7) Consultants should hold out-patient clinics at small local hospitals whenever possible	23	21	10	8	5	2
(9) District nurses should also nurse patients in small local hospitals	10	28	13	10	3	5
(5) Surgical procedures undertaken in small local hospitals should not extend beyond those which GPS would expect to perform in their own practice premises or in a health centre	26	19	6	13	3	2
(3) The fear of hospitals felt by some elderly patients is often strong enough to impair the beneficial effect of hospital care	10	31	9	13	2	4
(10) In places where there is a small hospital the local group practice premises should be attached or in its grounds	7	14	32	8	5	3
(6) No delivery (maternity) facilities should be provided in small local hospitals	22	12	10	12	10	3
(12) Elderly patients with dementia should be looked after in small local hospitals which also have other types of patients	9	15	17	15	9	4

Table 3.13

General practitioners' attitudes to issues (in order of agreement)

Statement	Strongly Agree	Agree	Neither	Disagree	Strongly Disagree	No reply
(2) Patients derive benefit from care in hospitals near their homes where they can easily be visited and maintain their links with the community	34	32	2	0	0	2
(7) Consultants should hold out-patients clinics at small local hospitals whenever possible	27	35	5	0	0	3
(8) Greater efforts should be made to admit elderly patients to hospitals for short rather than long stays	30	33	3	0	0	4
(1) Small local hospitals seem less formal and forbidding to patients than larger hospitals	35	24	7	1	1	2
(4) Day to day medical care both of in-patients and day patients in small local hospitals should be provided by GPs	20	29	13	5	1	2
(3) The fear of hospitals felt by some elderly patients is often strong enough to impair the beneficial effects of hospital care	17	31	11	8	1	2
(11) No emergency or accident cases should be treated in a small local hospital other than those which would be dealt with in a GPs surgery	21	23	6	12	2	6
(9) District nurses should also nurse patients in small local hospitals	10	26	16	9	5	4
(10) In places where there is a small hospital the local group practice premises should be attached or in its grounds	7	17	27	9	6	4
(6) No delivery (maternity) facilities should be provided in small local hospitals	17	18	7	13	11	4
(5) Surgical procedures undertaken in small local hospitals should not extend beyond those which GPs would expect to perform in their own practice premises or in a health centre	15	17	7	20	7	4
(12) Elderly patients with dementia should be looked after in small local hospitals which also have other types of patients	5	15	14	23	9	4

The question of whether group practice premises should be attached to community hospitals also produced a sizeable minority who disagreed with the statement. However, perhaps the most significant feature of the answers on this issue is the high proportion in the "neither agree nor disagree" category, suggesting that this question may be too general to be useful.

The statement that no maternity delivery facilities should be provided in community hospitals also proved controversial. Although there was a small majority in agreement with the statement there was a substantial number against. Indeed, of all the issues, this produced the largest number of respondents stating that they strongly disagreed. Several GPs stressed that they believed a good standard of care would be possible in community hospitals. From the hospital doctors there were some comments that maternity delivery in community hospitals would be feasible where back-up facilities were available in the main obstetric unit and where there was co-operation between consultants and GPs. Of the eight specialists in obstetrics and gynaecology who answered this question, five strongly agreed, two disagreed and one strongly disagreed, thus closely reflecting the pattern of responses of hospitals doctors as a whole.

The only statement to attract more doctors in disagreement than in agreement was that elderly patients with dementia should be looked after in small local hospitals which also have other types of patient, although a frequently expressed view was of neither agreement nor disagreement. Amongst hospital doctors, views were very evenly balanced. Perhaps one reason for this and the high proportion of unsure respondents was that (as several doctors pointed out) it would depend very largely on the severity of the cases. Interestingly, the statement appears to have produced different responses from psychiatrists and geriatricians. Five out of eight psychiatrists were in favour, with only one psychiatrist in disagreement (because it would lead to blocked beds and so defeat one of the objects of the community hospital). In contrast, geriatricians were three to one against the idea. Apart from the comment that elderly patients with dementia would be a disturbance to other patients, the only other adverse comment was that it might not be possible to maintain the large numbers of staff required by such patients in a small local hospital. As it was, the statement prompted a balanced response from the hospital doctors. Amongst GPs, disagreement with the statement was rather greater. In fact, this was the only issue with which more GPs disagreed than agreed. Some GPs commented that it was desirable in principle but was likely to be rather difficult in practice. It was suggested by some that such patients would be disruptive for other patients, that staffing a hospital containing such patients might be difficult and that special nursing care would be required. As amongst the hospital doctors there were several comments that the desirability of this policy is very dependent on the severity of the condition and on the number of patients involved.

So far, the responses have been separated only into hospital doctors and general practitioners, but, as there may be significantly different responses between different types of doctor in each of these groups, further disaggregation is of interest. Amongst the hospital doctors, consultants might be separated from other doctors on the grounds that they are in positions of greater experience and influence and therefore their views are of more immediate concern. A further reason for examining the difference between the opinions of consultants and junior doctors is that this method is the only one available for heralding any shifts in attitude which may be expected in the future. Needless to say, to assume that junior doctors will retain the same views several years hence, after attaining consultant status, is extremely dubious, so the method can be used only very tentatively. In the event, however, when the sample was divided into consultants and junior doctors and the total number agreeing with a statement was compared with the total number disagreeing, very little difference was found. For ten of the statements, the views of consultants and junior doctors corresponded closely and a statistically significant difference was detected only in two cases (using the chi square test at the 0.05 significance level). The largest disagreement was on the maternity issue: consultants tended to favour the statement that there should be no delivery facilities in small local hospitals (23 for the statement, 7 against) while junior doctors tended to oppose this view (11 for, 15 against). This difference is large enough to be considered a real difference, unlikely to have been caused by chance, and might therefore be hypothesised to occur in other health districts. Whether it will persist into the future is very uncertain. Rather less (but still statistically significant) disagreement occurred over the emergency and accident statement. Both groups tended to agree with it, but junior doctors by a lower margin (consultants: 32 for, 3 against; junior doctors: 20 for, 9 against).

A similar test was also carried out to determine whether the views of consultants under 50 years old were different from those of consultants of 50 and over, but no significant differences were found in the reactions of the two groups to the twelve statements. Status and age therefore appear to have little effect on the attitudes of hospital doctors towards the policy.

Further analysis of the data on GPs showed that the pattern of responses did not generally differ significantly by age, the possession of higher qualifications, number of years in the present practice, the size of practice or list size. An exception to this was that GPs in practices with four or more partners were significantly more in agreement with the statement that group practices should be attached to community hospitals. They were also more likely to agree that elderly patients with dementia should be treated in community hospitals which also have other patients. Agreement with this statement was also greater for those GPs with larger NHS lists (2,500+). GPs in the rural areas were more likely to disagree with the view that district nurses should nurse patients in community hospitals. They were also more likely to disagree with the statement that group practices should be attached to these hospitals.

Bearing in mind these qualifications about particular sub-groups amongst general practitioners and hospital doctors, it is possible to draw some general conclusions about their attitudes to community hospital policy. The most important finding is that a majority of doctors, and on some issues a very large majority, agree with the major features of community hospital policy. However, on certain issues opinion is much more diverse. For example, there is likely to be considerable debate within the medical profession at district level as to whether community hospitals should have facilities for maternity delivery and for surgery, and whether they should contain elderly mentally infirm patients. Clearly, the final form that each community hospital takes will reflect the local debate and may diverge from the DHSS guidelines. But even though there is a wide measure of agreement in principle with the community hospital policy, this is not to say that the policy will necessarily be practicable. For community hospitals to be successful, the doctors' generally favourable response must be translated into the active involvement of GPs in staffing such hospitals and the willingness of consultants to hold out-patients clinics at them.

Hospital doctors views on in-patients in community hospitals

The community hospital policy does not imply a simple transfer of suitable patients from a general hospital to a community hospital as many people who at present are not in hospital could be admitted for short periods. Furthermore, in the long term, an orientation towards prevention in the health and social services could produce a rather different pattern of hospital admissions than exists now. For the foreseeable future, however, it seems reasonable to assume that broadly the same types of patient will continue to be admitted to the available hospital beds. A key question is: what proportion of patients presently under the care of a consultant and occupying a bed in a general hospital, with its ancillary services and facilities, could be equally well cared for in a simpler community hospital? In the survey, hospital doctors were asked what proportion of the in-patients for whom they were responsible could be adequately cared for in a small local hospital by a general practitioner. They were also asked to distinguish between those patients who could be looked after by a GP without direct consultant supervision and those where direct consultant supervision would be required. ("Direct consultant supervision" was not defined and was therefore open to the interpretation placed upon it by each respondent).

Even when broken down by specialty the answers to the two questions varied widely between doctors. Of the five geriatricians, for example, three replied 'none', one replied '20%' and one replied '70%' to the first question. The various estimates have been summarised by identifying the median (or "middle") consultant opinion in each specialty and using the views of junior doctors as a check. Table 3.14 gives the results. To preserve confidentiality, the estimates made by only one consultant in a specialty have been omitted from the table. Thus the estimates for chest diseases, dental surgery, dermatology, general medicine, geriatric medicine, orthopaedics, rheumatology and urology are not shown. ENT surgery is also not included in the table as no consultant opinion was available. Some of the estimates are considered less reliable than others. Those marked as being less reliable are in at least one of the following two categories:

(i)   The figure given is based on widely differing estimates - all estimates differed by more than 10%;

(ii) The consultants' median was not corroborated by the junior doctors' median - the two medians differed by more than 10%.

Table 3.14

Consultants' assessments of percentages of in-patients who could be treated in a small local hospital, by specialty

Specialty	% Patients without consultant	Additional % patients with consultant	Number of Consultants
General surgery	20	25*	2
Radiotherapy	15	25*	2
Obstetrics/Gynaecology	10	30	3
Psychiatry	10	10	5
Cardiology	5	10	2
Paediatrics	0	5	2
Opthalmology	0	0	2
Thoracic surgery	0	0	3

* less reliable estimate

Even the "more reliable" estimates in Table 3.14 must be treated with great caution as they are based on very few opinions. Of course it may be said that in any Health District the way patients in different specialties are allocated to beds in small hospitals is, and will continue to be, the result of a very few opinions, but the medians offer no clue to the range likely to be encountered within a specialty. An indication of the range is obtained by examining the 42 occasions when the estimates of more than one consultant in the same specialty can be compared with their median.

As Table 3.15 shows, over four fifths of the estimates did not differ from their medians by more than 10%. The remaining fifth contained substantial differences, including one difference of 40%. This need not be solely a measure of the differences in judgement between consultants, for it is also affected by the heterogeneity of patients in the same specialty. Each respondent was asked to make an estimate from his own current patients and we expect that consultants in the same specialty may well concentrate on patients with different characteristics. Table 3.15 provides another indication that Table 3.14 must be regarded simply as a tentative first estimate.

The first conclusion to be drawn from these results is that in the opinion of hospital doctors only a small proportion of their patients could be adequately cared for in a small local hospital without consultant supervision. Among the four specialties where estimates were made in excess of 10% (of which two have been excluded from the table), only surgery accounts for a large absolute number of patients. In most specialties the estimates were of 10% or under. Providing direct consultant supervision almost always increases the percentage of eligible patients (by the amount in the middle column of the table). Addition of the two percentages gives a notional total percentage of patients who would be deemed suitable for a small local hospital if consultant cover were available.

Table 3.15
Differences between consultant estimates and medians

Differences in estimates	Frequency	Percentage
0%	22	52
10%	13	31
20%	3	7
30%	3	7
40%	1	2

One way to place these percentages in perspective is to multiply them by the average daily bed occupancy (East Anglian Regional Health Authority, 1976) for the relevant specialty in the King's Lynn District. There are some problems in using bed occupancy rates for the district rather than the region as patient transfers across district boundaries mean that district bed allocations do not necessarily reflect the bed usages of people resident in the district. On the other hand, consultants in the King's Lynn District replied to the questionnaire on the basis of the patients who were under their care, so on the whole it seems safer not to amend the district daily bed occupation rates. As the district has no beds listed under cardiology, radiotherapy, and thoracic surgery these specialties have been omitted. Table 3.16 gives for each specialty which has information available the average daily bed occupancy during 1975 in the King's Lynn District and this figure multiplied by the percentages of patients considered eligible for a small local hospital, both without and with consultant super-vision. Since the patients who could be suitably cared for without consultant supervision would still be eligible if such supervision were provided, they are now included in the last column.

If Table 3.14 needs to be treated with caution, the same is doubly true of Table 3.16. Nevertheless, the message appears sufficiently strong to override the inaccuracy of its details. A rough estimate of the number of beds in the King's Lynn District which could be filled by patients in the care of GPs without consultant supervision has been derived from consultants' consideration of their hospital patients. It will be recalled that several specialties were omitted from Table 3.14 for reasons of confidentiality. If estimates for chest diseases, dental surgery, general medicine, geriatrics and orthopaedics are included, the total estimated daily bed occupation is 31.5 without consultant supervision and 148.9 with consultant super-vision. These numbers should be multiplied by a bed occupancy rate to give the estimated number of beds required. In comparison, accord-ing to the DHSS guidelines, the 1981 population of the King's Lynn District would warrant a maximum of about 260 community hospital beds - a figure which is an order of magnitude greater than the first estimate and almost twice the second estimate. The conclusion is that the only way to reconcile the community hospital policy with the views of most consultants is either to ensure that community hospitals serve a different type of patient from those at present in hospital, or to continue consultant cover in small local hospitals. This conclusion is reassuring in that it appears to confirm that the specialised attention is given to hospital patients is considered justified by consultants in the large majority of cases. In the short term, in a climate of financial stringency and bed shortages, it appears to argue against the conversion of small hospitals into wholly GP units.

Table 3.16
Approximate numbers of beds in small local hospitals by specialty

Specialty	Average daily bed occupation	Estimated daily bed occupation of eligible patients	
		without consultant	with consultant cover
General surgery	57.5	11.5	25.9
Obstetrics/Gynaecology	81.1	8.1	32.4
Psychiatry (Mental illness)	19.4	1.9	3.9
Paediatrics	9.0	0	0.5
Opthalmology	5.3	0	0
Other specialties	0	10.0	86.2
Totals		31.5	148.9

The proportions of patients consultants would be willing to see treated by a GP in a small hospital have been shown to be small. A little light can be thrown on the types of patients in this category by Table 3.17, which lists certain patient types in order of frequency of mention. Of the patients who are considered not to require consultant supervision, social admissions and terminal admissions appear to be the most common groups. These types of patients are less prominent among those who are thought to require consultant care in a small hospital, where patients undergoing rehabilitation and other patients not fitting the specific categories used were mentioned most frequently.

Table 3.17
Percentage of hospital doctors mentioning various patient types as being suitable for a small local hospital

Without consultant supervision		Additional patients with consultant supervision	
Patient type	% mentions	Patient type	% mentions
Social admissions	56	Undergoing rehabilitation	30
Terminal admissions	56	Other patients	30
Geriatric patients	35	Geriatric patients	27
Undergoing rehabilitation	30	Social admissions	27
Preconvalescents	23	Terminal admissions	25
Geriatric with dementia	14	Preconvalescents	25
Other patients	9	Geriatrics with dementia	22

Hospital doctors views on the devolution of out-patients clinics to community hospitals

It is part of the community hospital policy that out-patient clinics should be held in small local hospitals.   To find out which specialties are the most suitable and to get an approximate idea of how many patients could be involved in the King's Lynn District, hospital doctors were asked several questions on the topic.   The following analysis is based on the replies of the 49 hospital doctors who attended out-patient clinics.   Doctors were asked to estimate the proportion of their first attendance out-patients they could see satisfactorily in a community hospital with the following facilities: consulting room, examination room, clinical test room, reception office, patients' waiting room, straight x-ray facility, specimen collection service, pharmaceutical service and nursing and secretarial support.   They were then asked the same question with regard to out-patients who were re-attendances. Their replies have been summarised by taking the median estimate in each specialty and the results are given in Table 3.18.   Specialties in which only one opinion was available have been omitted from the table. These are anaesthetics, chest diseases, cytology, dental surgery, dermatology, pathology, thoracic surgery and urology.   The median estimates in the table are identified as being less reliable if they are based on estimates which all differ by more than 10%.

Table 3.18
Assessment of out-patients who could be seen in a community hospital, by specialty

Specialty	% First Attendances	% Re-attendances	Number of doctors
Psychiatry	100	100	6
General surgery	90	90	3
General medicine	80	80	3
Paediatrics	80	80	3
Obstetrics/Gynaecology	75	80	8
ENT	55*	55*	2
Geriatric medicine	55*	55*	2
Radiotherapy	50*	65*	2
Rheumatology	20	20	2
Orthopaedics	10	30*	3
Cardiology	0	5	2
Opthalmology	0	0	3

* less reliable estimate

The use of the median estimates is a convenient way of summarising the views offered, but it does hide a considerable variation in the individual returns.   For all the specialties where more than one opinion was available, Table 3.19 shows the distribution of differences between individual estimates and medians and reveals that these estimates are much more variable that those for in-patients.   Only 56% of individual estimates were within 10% of the median which represented

them.   Two thirds of the individuals were within 20% of the median,
but for the remaining third the medians are hardly representative.

Table 3.19
Differences between individual estimates and medians in Table 3.18

Differences	Frequency	Percentage
0%	28	36
1 - 10%	16	21
11 - 20%	8	10
21 - 50%	19	24
51 -100%	7	9

A total of 9% of the estimates were more than 50% removed from the
medians.   These differences occured in the following specialties:
obstetrics and gynaecology, opthalmology and psychiatry.   The medians
in these three specialties are not considered particularly open to
doubt as all contained a majority of doctors who agreed closely with
the medians.   The message of Table 3.19, however, is that because of
large differences in estimates the information contained in Table 3.18
is an inaccurate guide.   Nonetheless, it is a guide where previously
no guide existed.

For some specialties, the percentages given in Table 3.18 might be
underestimates.   When asked to list additional facilities that would
substantially increase the proportions, paediatricians mentioned
physiotherapy, the services of a medical social worker, someone to
take blood samples and telephone contact with colleagues at the main
hospital.   Psychiatrists mentioned EEG and psychology services and
facilities for a psychotherapist, social worker and physiotherapist.
Specialists in general medicine mentioned an ECG machine and obstetricians an ultrasound machine and transport to the main hospital.
A plaster room with appropriate staff, bandage and dressings facilities
and physiotherapy were listed by orthopaedics specialists, and physiotherapy, occupational therapy, a social worker and dressing facilities
by rheumatologists.   It is anticipated that many of these facilities
could be provided in a community hospital.   Other facilities which
were mentioned seem unlikely to be available outside the main hospital.
These include diagnostic X-ray facilities (medicine) a dental surgery
operating theatre, full urgent pathology and X-ray (radiotherapy),
opthalmic equipment, audiometry (ENT) and day surgery facilities
(general surgery).

The estimates of out-patients are more variable than those of in-
patients, but they are also noticeably higher.   To gain an idea of the
magnitude of the numbers involved, the annual out-patient attendances
in the King's Lynn District (East Anglian Regional Health Authority,
1976) have been multiplied by the percentages in Table 3.18, and the
products, representing estimates of the annual number of out-patient
attendances in each specialty which could be held in community
hospitals with simple facilities, are given in Table 3.20.

61

Table 3.20

Approximate numbers of out-patient attendances in community hospitals, by specialty

Specialty	Annual number of first attendances in District	Possible community hospital first attendance	Annual number of re-attend-ances in District	possible community hospital re-attendance
General surgery	3,780	3,402	10,303	9,273
Obstetrics/Gynaecology	4,210	3,157	11,828	9,462
ENT	1,798	989	2,902	1,596
Psychiatry	704	704	2,938	2,938
General medicine	672	538	3,142	2,514
Paediatrics	611	489	2,416	1,933
Orthopaedics	3,114	311	7,013	2,014
Geriatric medicine	254	140	545	300
Radiotherapy	140	70	2,558	1,663
Rheumatology	225	45	1,103	221
Cardiology	25	0	91	5
Opthalmology	1,645	0	5,643	0

When the omitted estimates for chest diseases, dental surgery, derma-tology, thoracic surgery and urology are added to the estimates in Table 3.20, the number of first attendances which are assessed as suitable for a community hospital with basic facilities amounts to 51% of the total first attendances in the district. Of the total re-attendances in the district, 57% are estimated to be suitable for community hospitals. It must again be stressed that these figures are merely indications, but they appear to be the only indications available.

By a very wide margin, the specialties with most out-patients who may be appropriately seen in a community hospital are general surgery and obstetrics/gynaecology. Some way behind, but still numbering suitable out-patients in the thousands, are ENT, general medicine, psychiatry, paediatrics, orthopaedics, radiotherapy and one of the omitted specialties.

Taking the four specialties with the largest totals of possible community hospital attendances in Table 3.20 (general surgery, obstet-rics/gynaecology, psychiatry and general medicine) the annual numbers of clinic sessions that might be held in community hospitals were calculated by dividing possible attendances by the average attendances per clinic session (East Anglian Regional Health Authority, 1976). The number of sessions per year were 453, 994, 1012 and 218 respectively. Even general medicine, with the smallest number of possible annual sessions, would therefore seem to be able to support a weekly clinic (an average of 54 clinic sessions per year) in no less than four community hospitals. The possible community hospital attendances in these four specialties alone account for 39% of the district's total out-patient attendances. Rounding this percentage, we conclude that, if numbers were the only consideration, at least 40% of the district's out-patient attendances could be made to viable decentralised clinics.

Numbers, of course, are not the only consideration. The other relevant factors are best discussed by summarising the advantages and disadvantages mentioned by respondents of holding out-patient clinics in small hospitals away from the general hospital. Of all the factors described, considerations related to travel predominate on both sides of the argument. A large number of doctors mentioned the reduced travelling time and costs for patients as an advantage of dispersed clinics and the increased travel time and costs of consultants as a disadvantage. Against the advantage of less working time lost for patients in a decentralised system must be set the reduced work load of consultants, with less patients seen and less opportunity for training junior doctors.

The second most frequently mentioned group of advantages were those deriving from the closer contact small hospitals have with the community. Small units were thought to be more personal and less intimidating for patients. Patients can also more easily bring friends or relatives for support to a local clinic than to a distant hospital. On the other hand, anonymity (which may be desirable in a minority of cases) is less easy to guarantee. Another advantage recognised by several hospital doctors is that dispersed clinics would improve their communications with GPs and add interest and satisfaction for the GPs themselves. In smaller clinics there would be shorter sessions and fewer patients, who could be examined more thoroughly and followed up more closely than at the general hospital - presumably at the expense of a higher work load overall.

On the negative side of the argument, the difficulty of working with incomplete facilities was mentioned several times. Careful selection of patients by the GP could reduce this disadvantage but some patients would inevitably have to make an additional journey to the main centre. Some doctors were concerned that dispersed clinics would cause professional contacts between colleagues and access to information services such as libraries and laboratories to be diminished, which might create a sense of isolation, as well as reducing the number of occasions when a problem could be resolved on the spot. Dispersed clinics may also cause consultants to be absent from the main centre on occasions when their services are required in an emergency. Others mentioned that dispersed clinics may need more supervision from consultants than clinics in the general hospital as the quality of staff might not be so high. Records would need to be duplicated or moved around and secretarial work would be increased. Two respondents were concerned that if out-patient facilities were close to people's homes this would increase the referral rate for conditions which could be dealt with by GPs in the community.

Examining the responses as a whole, the advantages and disadvantages of dispersed clinics appear to be finely balanced, but individual doctors tended to come down on one side or the other of the argument. When asked whether they agreed with the principle of holding decentralised clinics for their own specialties, 27 said yes, 17 said no, and 4 did not know. The breakdown by specialty is given in Table 3.21. Again, specialties with only one respondent have been omitted. This information indicates that in the King's Lynn District a clear majority of doctors in the two specialties which would be the most viable in terms of patient numbers (general surgery and obstetrics/gynaecology)

63

favoured the decentralisation of clinics.   In other specialties which
appear to be able to supply large numbers of outpatients (psychiatry,
medicine, ENT, orthopaedics and geriatric medicine) hospital doctors
appear to be less enthusiastic, although paediatrics and radiotherapy
produced unanimous views in favour.   The key question is, of course,
to what extent is approval of the idea of decentralised clinics a
function of the specialty and to what extent is it governed by personal
factors (which might well cause a different pattern of views in another
district)?   In an attempt to answer this, agreement with decentralised
clinics was compared with a number of attributes: grade, age, the
number of clinics attended by the doctor, and the doctor's assessment
of the proportion of patients in his specialty who could be seen at a
decentralised clinic.   Of these, only the last factor was found to be
significant at the 0.05 level with a chi square test.   Assessments of
percentages of out-patients who could appropriately be seen at a local
clinic have been divided into those less than 50% and those of 50% and
over (Table 3.22).   It can be seen both for first attendances and re-
attendances that respondents who make high estimates are more likely to
be in agreement with decentralised clinics (or perhaps vice versa).
When the "don't know" responses are omitted, a chi square test gives a
significant difference at the 0.01 level.

Table 3.21
Agreement with decentralised clinics, by specialty

Specialty	Yes	No	Don't know
Cardiology	1	1	0
ENT surgery	0	2	0
Geriatric medicine	1	1	0
General medicine	2	1	0
Obstetrics/Gynaecology	6	1	1
Opthalmology	1	1	1
Orthopaedics	2	1	0
Paediatrics	3	0	0
Psychiatry	3	4	1
Rheumatology	0	2	0
Radiotherapy	2	0	0
Surgery	3	0	0

As the out-patient percentage estimates are correlated with the
estimated out-patient numbers in Table 3.20 it is not surprising that
the specialties which seem to be able to produce most out-patients
suitable for decentralised clinics also produce most doctors in agreement with the policy.   Similarly, doctors in the specialties where only
small numbers of patients would be involved tend to be against the policy
(Table 3.23, the dividing line has been arbitrarily taken at 1,000
total attendances).   Again omitting the "don't know" category, the
association is statistically significant at the 0.01 level.

Table 3.22

Agreement with decentralised clinics, by out-patient estimates

	Yes	No	Don't know
First attendances			
less than 50%	5	11	2
50-100%	22	6	1
Re-attendances			
less than 50%	4	12	2
50-100%	23	5	1

To summarise, opinions on the issue of whether clinics should be decentralised are not affected by grade, age or the number of clinics attended, but they are quite strongly affected by the doctor's assessment of the number of patients who could benefit from the arrangement.

Table 3.23

Agreement with decentralised clinics with estimated total attendances

	Yes	No	Don't know
less than 1,00 attendances	4	10	2
more than 1,000 attendances	23	7	2

STAFFING PROBLEMS

No matter how desirable community hospitals are in principle they will not be feasible unless they can attract sufficient qualified staff. Two main groups of personnel are likely to be of particular importance. general practitioners willing to undertake the daily medical care of patients in community hospitals; and nurses, physiotherapists, occupational therapists and radiographers. The surveys collected information on the likelihood of community hospitals being able to attract each of these groups. Discussion with administrators in the King's Lynn District suggested that the recruitment of other ancillary hospital staff would probably pose few difficulties and therefore such staff were not investigated.

The willingness of general practitioners to participate in community hospitals

The development of community hospitals in the form suggested by the DHSS will require the active involvement of GPs in the area where the hospital is located. A major question about any proposed site for a community hospital is whether there are sufficient GPs in the vicinity willing to undertake the day to day medical care of in-patients and

perhaps to be on call for emergencies. Does this type of work fit
in with the career aspirations of many general practitioners? What
proportion are interested in working in community hospitals and how far
would they be prepared to travel? The results of the survey of
general practitioners allow some conclusions to be drawn on these
questions.

Table 3.24 suggests that the development of community hospitals
would fit in with the career aspirations of some GPs. The respondents
were asked in what direction they would wish to develop interests in
the future, assuming they were able to make the necessary time available.
It seems that about half the GPs who responded to this question would
be interested in the type of hospital work which an appointment in a
community hospital could offer and, on the other hand, about half would
not. The fact that a substantial minority did not answer all parts of
the question, however, suggests that the question is not a reliable
measure.

Table 3.24
Development of GPs' interests in the future

	Very Interested	Interested	Not Interested
Working solely as a GP	34	22	5
Special clinical interests in hospital	26	17	17
Care of hospital in-patients after surgery	7	23	30
Care of geriatric patients in hospital	6	28	25
Care of social cases in hospital	1	27	32
Care of hospital day patients	2	22	33
Work in school and pre-school clinics	7	6	40

More specific information on the likely problems of staffing a
community hospital was obtained by asking the GPs surveyed whether, in
principle, they felt they would like to participate in a community
hospital.

Table 3.25
Willingness to participate in a community hospital

Willingness	Number
Definitely yes	32
Possibly yes	27
Unlikely	8
Definitely not	1

Table 3.25 demonstrates a high level of interest in participation.
Only one doctor said he definitely would not wish to participate and a
relatively small number said they were unlikely to do so.   On the other
hand approximately 47% of those answering this question said they would
definitely wish to participate and a further 40% said that they might
wish to participate in a community hospital.   Factors such as age, the
possession of higher qualifications, the number of years spent in the
present practice, the size of the practice, and whether the practice
was urban or rural had no significant effect (at the 0.05 level).
Thus it appears that, in principle at least, a fairly high proportion
of GPs in the King's Lynn District would probably be willing to work in
a community hospital.   The prospects of finding doctors to staff such
hospitals in the district therefore seem to be fairly good.   However,
the question asked of the GPs was whether in principle they were
prepared to participate.   In practice, the situation might be different.
Numerous comments made by the doctors suggests that to attract GPs to
work in community hospitals it will be necessary for them to be adequately paid and for their existing work loads to be reduced.   It is
interesting in this connection to report that general practitioners
working in the Peppard Hospital, the original community hospital pilot,
spent an average of only 3.2 hours in the ward each week, and this was
to some extent balanced by a reduction in home visiting (Hasler, 1974).

In addition to pay and work load it is also likely that a large number
of other factors will affect whether GPs are willing to work in a
community hospital.   Two such factors, the distance of the community
hospital from the GP's home and whether a doctor is on call for a minor
accident service in the hospital, were investigated because they were
felt to be of particular importance.

Table 3.26

GPs' interest in working in a community hospital at different
distances from home

Distance from home	Very Interested	Interested	Not Interested
0 - 5 miles	36	25	4
5 - 10 miles	10	20	37
over 10 miles	4	9	50

Table 3.27

Percentage of urban and rural GPs who are very interested or
interested in participating in a community hospital related to
distance

	0-5 miles	5-10 miles	Over 10 miles
Urban GPs	100	25	5
Rural GPs	91	57	29

Table 3.26 shows that most GPs would be prepared to travel up to five miles. However, 55% would not be prepared to work in a community hospital between five and ten miles from their home whilst 79% would not be prepared to participate if this involved travelling more than ten miles. So far as GP involvement is concerned, the catchment areas of community hospitals are likely to be geographically rather small. This suggests that a community hospital located where there are few GPs living close by is likely to experience difficulties in attracting sufficient numbers of them to participate in it. However, Table 3.27 suggests that GPs in the rural areas might be prepared to travel further than those in urban areas. If this is a general phenomenon, greater willingness to travel may be expected to counteract the staffing difficulties which might otherwise exist in rural areas where GPs are geographically rather thinly spread.

Table 3.28
GPs' interest in working in a community hospital involving periods of being on call for a minor accident service

Distance from home	Very Interested	Interested	Not Interested
0 - 5 miles	28	24	12
5 - 10 miles	9	14	42
Over 10 miles	4	4	53

A comparison of Tables 3.26 and 3.28 shows that the existence of a minor accident service in a community hospital requiring GPs to be on call would be likely to reduce the numbers who would be interested in working in the hospital. The extent of this reduction is fairly small, though. For example, 94% of respondents said they would be interested in working in a community hospital less than 5 miles away and without a minor accident service, but with an accident service this was reduced to 81%. Similar reductions apply for other distances. It therefore seems that the presence of a minor accident service requiring GPs to be on call would have a small but measurable effect on the ease with which GPs could be persuaded to co-operate in the staffing of a community hospital.

The attitudes of nurses, physiotherapists, occupational therapists and radiographers to work in a community hospital

In many ways, working in a community hospital will be rather different from working in other types of hospital. The mix of patients treated in such hospitals will not be the same as elsewhere. Community hospitals will also be rather smaller than most staff members have been used to and, whereas most large hospitals are in the main towns, many community hospitals will be located in smaller places. Some of these features will be attractive to potential staff whilst others will act as deterrents. There is therefore the possibility that it may be difficult to attract the key groups of nurses, physiotherapists, occupational therapists and radiographers in sufficient numbers to work in community hospitals.

Much of the work in community hospitals will involve unspectacular
(although skillful) care of patients, many of them with chronic ill-
nesses.   In particular, there will be a high proportion of elderly
patients, some of them perhaps mentally infirm.   There is therefore
clearly a question of whether this type of work will be attractive to
trained staff.   This question was explored by identifying the types
of patient likely to be encountered in a community hospital and asking
staff how interested they were in working with each type.   The results
are given in Table 3.29.

Table 3.29
Preferences for working with different types of patients

Patient type		Very Interested	Interested	Not Interested	Don't know or not applic- able
Geriatric	% nurses	29	45	15	11
	% other staff	10	53	27	10
Preconva- lescent	% nurses	33	45	10	12
	% other staff	17	33	33	17
Physically handicapped	% nurses	11	33	29	27
	% other staff	27	37	23	13
Elderly with dementia	% nurses	7	30	37	26
	% other staff	3	13	70	13
Terminal	% nurses	28	46	13	13
	% other staff	3	20	43	33

The attractiveness of a hospital containing at least some of the above
patient groups for nurses, occupational therapists, physiotherapists
and radiographers is a complex issue touching upon such things as the
proportions of the various groups, the extent of physical handicap,
the degree to which an elderly patient suffers dementia and the context
of the care that a patient receives.   The format of the question
presented to staff in the survey ignores these complexities.   Nevertheless, the replies appear to indicate marked differences in the attitudes
held by staff to the various patient groups.   Taking nursing staff
alone, around three quarters of all nurses expressed some interest
(by ticking the "very interested" or "interested" categories) in the
care of geriatric, preconvalescent and terminal patients.   The
corresponding proportion for physically handicapped patients was just
under half, and a little over a third of nurses in the survey expressed
an interest in working with elderly patients suffering from dementia
(it will be recalled from the surveys of hospital doctors and general
 practitioners that there is some doubt whether such patients are suitable for community hospitals).   We conclude that the types of patients
likely to be found in a community hospital are not likely to substantially discourage the recruitment of trained nurses.

69

Although physiotherapists, occupational therapists and radiographers were markedly less enthusiastic than the nurses about the types of patients mentioned (with the exception of the physically handicapped), a majority of them were either interested or very interested in working with geriatric patients, preconvalescent patients and physically handicapped patients. This is not to say, of course, that a majority would necessarily be happy to work exclusively with these groups, but looked at simply from the point of view of staff preferences for patient type, the problem of finding physiotherapists, occupational therapists and radiographers to serve such patients is not likely to be insuperable. Patients in the terminal stage and especially mentally infirm elderly patients were much less "popular" among the non-nursing trained staff surveyed. Certainly a job which consisted almost entirely of working with these two types of patient (if such a job could be conceived) would be difficult to fill, judging by the responses reported here. The answer would appear to lie in providing physiotherapists, occupational therapists and radiographers with as wide a variety of work as possible.

The next question to be explored is whether the smallness of community hospitals is likely to deter staff. This issue was approached by presenting nurses and other groups of staff with a list of sixteen possible factors concerned with hospital work. Respondents were asked to indicate how important each of these was to them in terms of job satisfaction, using a three point scale, and also to indicate whether each factor was more often found in a large or a small hospital.

To express the comparative importance of each of the factors, they have been ranked in order of the percentage of respondents marking either the "very important" or "important" categories. When this was done for nurses and non-nursing staff separately the two lists were very similar, with the most important factors (friendly relationships with hospital staff, flexibility and variety of work, and work which makes full use of training and experience) and the least important factors (the social life of the hospital and the opportunity to live in) occupying identical positions in both lists. The correlation coefficient between the two lists (in terms of the percentage responses in the important and very important categories) was 0.93. This indicates a very strong relationship between the comparative importance of the factors for nursing and non-nursing staff. The factors are arranged in Table 3.30, in descending order of job satisfaction importance for the sample as a whole. The table is made up of the answers of each respondent to two questions. It reveals how each factor is viewed both in terms of job satisfaction importance and whether it is thought to be associated with large or small hospitals. Numbers are raw responses, not percentages.

Although substantial proportions of respondents chose the central category "not related to size of hospital" for almost all the factors, equally substantial proportions distinguished some factors as being characteristic of large hospitals (defined as over 300 beds) and some as being found more often in small hospitals (of less than 50 beds). On most factors, nurses and non-nursing staff were in broad agreement but there was a slight tendency for non-nursing staff generally to associate factors important for job satisfaction with large hospitals compared with nursing staff. This can be seen in Table 3.31, where the replies relating to all factors are pooled together. Large and small hospitals received an almost equal number of nurses' votes in the "very important" category, while large hospitals were favoured more by non-nursing staff.

Table 3.30
Factors relating job satisfaction and hospital size

	Hospital size associated with factor:	Large	Unrelated	Small
(n) Friendly relations with all hospital staff with whom you work regularly	Very important	1	37	38
	Important	0	20	18
	Not important	0	0	0
(c) Flexibility and variety in work	Very important	33	22	9
	Important	12	29	7
	Not important	1	0	0
(j) Work which makes full use of training and experience	Very important	33	36	8
	Important	8	23	2
	Not important	1	1	0
(o) Each member feeling that his contribution is valued by other members of the hospital staff	Very important	0	49	30
	Important	1	21	9
	Not important	0	4	0
(i) Working with experienced and skilled hospital staff	Very important	32	34	0
	Important	19	25	0
	Not important	1	4	0
(k) Opportunities to increase training and experience	Very important	45	16	0
	Important	31	12	0
	Not important	9	0	0
(e) A lot of contact with hospital doctors	Very important	7	20	11
	Important	16	28	17
	Not important	4	8	3
(a) A wide variety of types of patients to care for	Very important	33	20	2
	Important	20	19	2
	Not important	5	11	0
(h) Use of and experience with the most modern equipment	Very important	30	10	0
	Important	48	6	0
	Not important	13	4	1
(b) Being able to get to know patients personally	Very important	0	21	35
	Important	0	15	24
	Not important	0	6	13
(d) Plenty of information on the home circumstances of patients	Very important	0	16	22
	Important	3	28	22
	Not important	0	10	10

Table 3.30
Factors relating job satisfaction and hospital size

	Hospital size associated with factor:	Large	Unrelated	Small
(1) Personal preferences for desirable working hours and time off taken into account	Very important	1	17	11
	Important	5	29	20
	Not important	3	19	5
(g) A lot of contact with the district nurses who will care for discharged patients	Very important	0	9	14
	Important	1	30	22
	Not important	0	21	13
(f) A lot of contact with the general practitioners of patients	Very important	1	1	15
	Important	0	16	32
	Not important	1	20	28
(m) The social life of the hospital	Very important	2	3	0
	Important	17	18	4
	Not important	38	27	4
(p) The opportunity to live in	Very important	1	4	0
	Important	4	4	1
	Not important	35	63	3

Apart from this distinction, there was a high level of agreement between nurses and other staff. The factors that were widely thought to be characteristic of large hospitals were flexibility and variety in work, work which makes full use of training and experience, working with experienced and skilled staff, opportunities to increase training and experience, a wide variety of patient types, use of the most modern equipment, a hospital social life and the opportunity to live in. Small hospitals were thought to be distinguished by friendly staff relations, a feeling that a person's work is valued by other staff members, the opportunity to get to know patients personally and to obtain information on patients' home circumstances, the likelihood of contact with district nurses and general practitioners and the possibility of having personal preferences for working hours taken into account.

All factors but two were considered to be important for job satisfaction by a majority of respondents. Since the respondents were all trained staff and many of them were married, it is not surprising that the social life of the hospital and the opportunity to live in were thought unimportant by most. Of the fourteen important factors, six were thought to be associated with large hospitals and seven with small hospitals. The difficulty with this sort of accounting procedure is, of course, that it is highly dependent on the factors that were selected by the investigators to be included in the questionnaire in the first place. The only firm conclusion possible is that both very large and very small hospitals are recognised as having their own advantages and neither is regarded as superior to the other by nurses, although members of the other occupational groups tended to favour large hospitals. A prominent characteristic of Table 3.31, is the large number of respondents who thought that almost all the important factors were not related to hospital size.   On the basis of this evidence it seems unlikely that there is a prejudice against small hospitals which could adversely affect staffing.

Table 3.31
Job satisfaction and hospital size : all factors

	Hospital size associated with factors:	Large	Unrelated	Small
Nurses	Very important	143	228	147
	Important	146	231	142
	Not important	90	133	57
Physiotherapists, occupational therapists and radiographers	Very important	76	87	48
	Important	39	87	36
	Not important	21	65	23

The answers to the question: "Which size of hospital would you prefer to work in?" are given in Table 3.32.   The most popular size of hospital for both groups was between 100 and 300 beds.   However, physio-therapists, occupational therapists and radiographers were more markedly in favour of the 100-300 bed size than nurses.   There is also a conspicuous absence of any physiotherapists, occupationsl therapists and radiographers among those who preferred hospitals in the two small-est categories.   When the size categories in Table 3.32 are collapsed into "small" (less than 100 beds), "large" (more than 100 beds) and "no preference" to enable a chi square test to be carried out, the difference between nurses and the other groups is significant at the 0.05 level.   We therefore expect this to be a real difference which exists outside our sample.

Table 3.32
Hospital size preference by professional groups

Size	% Nurses	% Other Groups
Less than 50 beds	5	0
Between 50 and 99 beds	11	0
Between 100 and 300 beds	38	55
More than 300 beds	7	16
No preference	39	29
BASE	84	31

Of those expressing a preference for a particular size of hospital,
87% had worked in a hospital of that size (not surprisingly, respondents
felt unwilling to express a preference for a type of hospital of which
they had no experience).   Since the sample contained people who, in
general, had more experience of hospitals with more than 100 beds we
might expect a general tendency to prefer larger hospitals.

Table 3.33
Experience and preference for hospital size

Hospital size	Worked in this size of hospital %	Worked in this size of hospital and preferred it %	preferred other %	no preference %
Less than 50 beds	34	8	49	41
50 to 99 beds	42	12	54	31
100 to 300 beds	76	50	18	31
More than 300 beds	60	13	48	38
BASE	115			

Column 1 of Table 3.33 shows the proportions of respondents who had
experience in hospitals in each size category and columns 2 to 4 show
the preferences of all those with any experience in a particular size
of hospital.   From the evidence of this table, the preference for a
hospital of 100-300 beds becomes more convincing.   Considerably more
people had worked in this size of hospital and preferred it than any
other size.

The final question to be considered is whether the location of
community hospitals in small market towns will create staffing problems.
One of the arguments in favour of such hospitals is that they will be
able to make use of local pools of trained staff who are not prepared
to travel large distances to work in a district general hospital.
If such reserves are not available community hospitals will have to
draw on the pool of people already employed in the health service.

The evidence of the survey is that nurses and the other categories of
staff investigated are a very mobile group.   Figure 3.1 shows that the
existing hospitals in the King's Lynn District are able to draw on
staff from a wide area.   This is confirmed by Table 3.34, showing the
distances travelled to work.   Although the majority of work trips (68%)
are less than 5 miles in length, this is not a disproportionate number
as approximately 65% of the health district's total population lives
within 5 miles of at least one of the hospitals.   The remaining work
trips are distributed over relatively long distances, with 20% of them
exceeding 10 miles.   The use of the private car for the journey to
work by 75% of the sample provides additional evidence of a highly
mobile group.

On the basis of this evidence it can be concluded that hospital staff
in the study area are prepared to travel fairly long distances to work
and that community hospitals would be able to draw on fairly wide

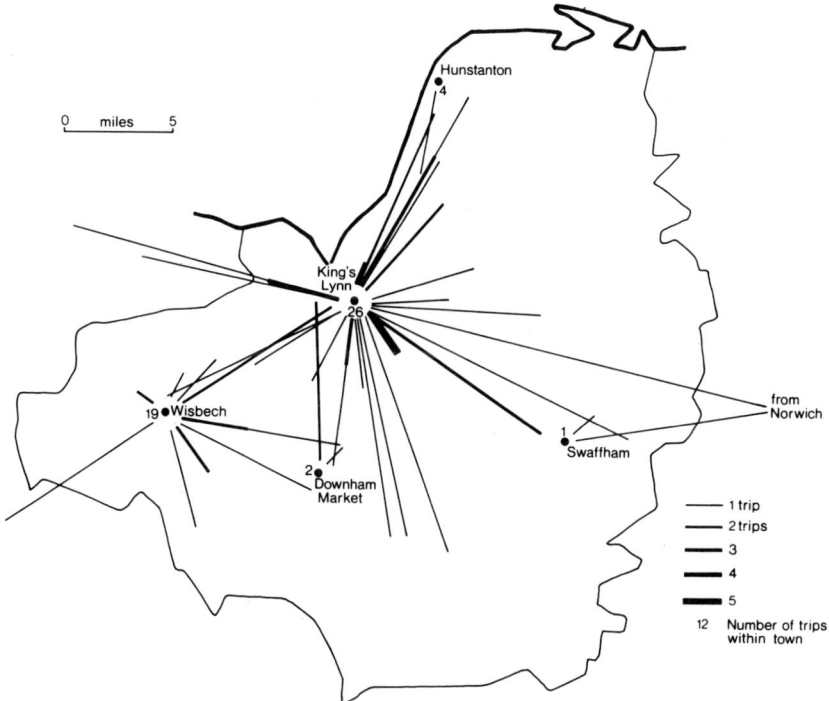

Figure 3.1   Work trips of nurses and other staff

Table 3.34
Journey to work distances

Mileage	%	Cumulative %
less than 5 miles	68	68
5-10 miles	12	80
10-15 miles	14	94
15-20 MILES	4	98
More than 20 miles	2	100
BASE	114	

catchment areas for staff.   This evidence, coupled with that of a
national survey (Sadler and Whitworth, 1975) which found that marriage
and children (and not distance) were the main factors which kept non-
active trained staff out of work, suggests that there is not a substantial reserve of trained staff in Norfolk which would be brought back
into service if a policy of small local hospitals were pursued.
However, the high mobility of hospital staff already living in the
district suggests that this need not be a barrier to the staffing of
community hospitals located in the market towns of the district.
Furthermore, our survey revealed that 30% of'the sample had moved into
the area specifically to take up or seek hospital employment, suggesting that community hospitals might be able to draw on an extremely wide

pool of labour.

THE COSTS OF COMMUNITY HOSPITALS

No matter how many advantages community hospitals might have, if they
are too expensive community hospital policy is unlikely to succeed.
Therefore, further crucial questions facing the planners of such
hospitals are how much are they likely to cost and how do these costs
compare with other ways of dealing with the patients involved?   Any
health authority embarking on a programme of community hospitals needs
to produce precise answers to these questions for the particular
developments proposed.   This study makes no attempt to produce such
costings for the community hospital strategies that might be applied
to the King's Lynn District.   This would require precise specifications
of the capital works that would be required and the way in which the
hospitals would be run.   Clearly many of the costs would be dependent
on particular local circumstances, for instance, whether extensions
to existing buildings are possible, and these would lack general
applicability.   Therefore, the approach of this study has been to
concentrate on the generalisations that can be made about the costs of
community hospitals.

It is conventional to distinguish two main categories of cost, capital
costs and revenue costs.   Each of these will be dealt with in turn.

Capital costs

The major elements of the capital costs of hospitals are the costs of
the land for the hospital, site development costs, the costs of building and equipping the wards and the costs of ancilliary services.

What can be concluded about the capital costs of community hospitals
as compared with the capital costs of an equivalent amount of provision
in a district general hospital?   Furthermore, what is known about the
variation in capital costs of community hospitals according to size and
location of hospital?   Rickard (1976) provides some general information
on these issues, based largely on a study of the estimated costs of
community hospitals in Wallingford and Witney.

Land costs will depend on the cost per acre of the land and on how
much land is used.   Assuming all sites have to be purchased (not a
realistic assumption since it is likely that the NHS will have sites
available or not fully utilised) the costs per acre of land should be
lower in small towns than in the larger towns and cities.   However,
Rickard shows that in the cases of Wallingford and Witney hospitals
the extensive use of land in low density development offsets much of
the apparent saving from lower unit costs of land.   Therefore much
will depend on the policies on the type of buildings to be built which
will influence the intensity of use of the site.

For the ward costs of new hospitals the DHSS issues guidance to
Regional Health Authorities in the form of detailed cost and area
allowances which must not be exceeded.   Rickard used these guidelines
to estimate what the cost of a district general hospital equivalent to
the community hospital he studied would have been.   He showed that by

building to a more domestic standard (essentially by allowing less space per patient) significant cost savings were possible. For example, the actual tender cost for phase 1 of the Wallingford Hospital was £112,000, whereas the calculated costs for equivalent provision in a district general hospital was £132,800 (January 1971 prices). Taking figures for Wallingford phase 1 and 2 together, Rickard estimated that comparing the community hospital with the district general hospital alternative there was a ward cost reduction of £550 per bed. (However, this depends on the DGH ward being built to a higher standard than the community hospital. If this is not the case the cost difference disappears).

Supporting service costs cover the costs of kitchens, boilers, etc. The level of these costs will depend critically on whether any existing supporting services have spare capacity. If not, addition of extra support services to a district general hospital ought to cost about the same as for a community hospital. However, if there are economies of scale in the provision of these services this conclusion would not be valid - costs would be lower in the larger district general hospital. Rickard suggests that it is difficult to find evidence for economies of scale. It therefore seems reasonable to assume that the capital costs for supporting services should not differ between district general hospital and community hospital alternatives, unless the district general hospital has spare capacity.

Revenue costs

It is possible to divide revenue costs into three main categories: ward costs, treatment costs and general services such as catering and laundry. There is a farily extensive literature which attempts to measure the main determinants of revenue costs. In particular, a number of studies have attempted to demonstrate the way in which revenue costs vary with hospital size and thereby specify the size of hospital which minimises costs (Carr and Feldstein, 1967; Feldstein, 1967; Berry, 1967; Cohen, 1967; Ro, 1968; Rickard, 1976). The most common approach in these studies is to analyse average cost data (cost per in-patient week or cost per case) and to attempt to explain variation in terms of hospital size, case mix, etc.. Usually regression analysis is the method used. Unfortunately many of these studies deal with larger, mainly acute hospitals and therefore their results are not particularly relevant to this study. Furthermore, the findings of the analyses have mostly been rather disappointing. The levels of explanation achieved by the regression models have generally been very low and the estimates of the least-cost size of hospitals have varied markedly from one study to another.

Rickard's study is the most relevant for community hospitals. He analysed data on the average costs of about 500 small (less than 100 beds) hospitals. Part of his sample (43 hospitals) were hospitals with mainly GP beds and without operating theatres, that is, hospitals which approximate to some of the characteristics of community hospitals. Average costs per bed (in 1970 figures) were regressed against number of beds. A quadratic function was found to give the best fit. Figure 3.2 gives the predicted values from the regression equation of average cost per bed for hospitals of different sizes. It shows that very

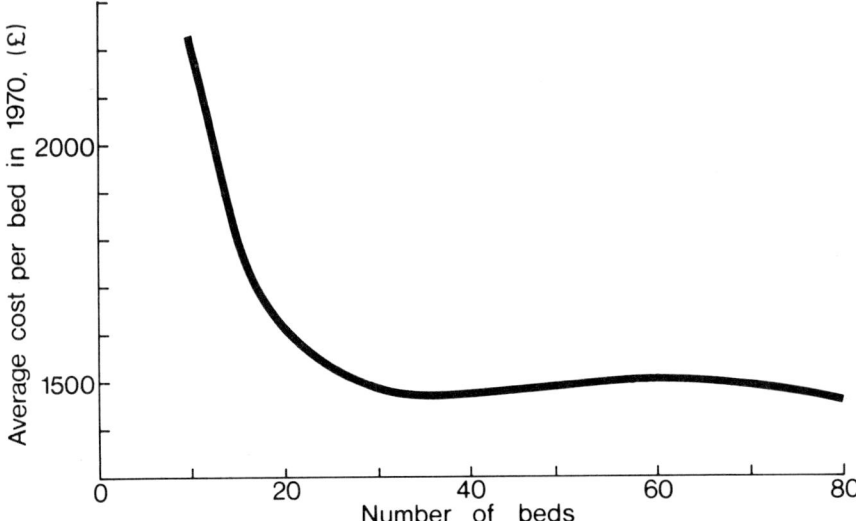

Figure 3.2   Average cost and hospital size (after Rickard)

small hospitals have rather high costs but that as size increases
average costs fall, reaching a minimum at 35 beds.   Above that size
(within the limits of the regression, that is, up to sizes of about
80 beds) there is little variation in cost with size.   If these find-
ints are relevant to community hospitals they suggest that hospitals
smaller than the size range set out in the DHSS community hospitals
circular would not incur revenue cost penalties except if they were less
than 35 beds.   This finding is clearly of potential importance where
it can be shown that more "social benefits" would accrue from a greater
number of small community hospitals than from a lesser number of
larger ones.

In addition to the general analysis of the costs of small hospitals
the Rickard study also calculates the revenue costs of the Wallingford
and Peppard Hospital community hospital wards.   The general conclusion
is that:

"... the community hospital wards, as they are at present
administered, are considerably more expensive than the DGH
alternative - the difference ranging from between 25% and 50%
more.   The reasons for this are the small scale of the two
experimental wards, the high level of nursing staff and, for
the transferred patient, the ambulance costs involved in the
transfer of patients."   (Rickard,   1976).

It seems likely that these findings will not be applicable to all
future community hospitals unless the rather lavish use of staff
characteristic of Wallingford is repeated, and there seems to be no
strong grounds for supposing that this will be the case.

The cost of domiciliary care

As well as comparing the costs of treatment in a district general
hospital and a community hospital it would also be necessary to consider
the costs of another alternative, that is, domiciliary care. The
costs of this to the NHS and to other agencies such as the social
services of local authorities can be estimated using a method developed
by Rickard. Briefly, this involves a number of elements:

(i)   Calculation of community nursing costs by a work study of a sample
      of these nurses. This would involve the calculation of costs
      per visit (salary plus travel) multiplied by the typical number
      of visits for a sample of patients with a similar nursing depend-
      ency to that expected for community hospital patients.

(ii) Calculation of costs per visit of home-helps, Meals on Wheels,
      etc., multiplied by the number of visits made.

(iii) Calculation of the costs of GP visits multiplied by the expected
      number of visits.

(iv) Calculation of the costs of drugs, etc.

As an example Rickard gives the following typical annual cost for
domiciliary care of someone in the top quartile of nursing dependency:

Nursing services	£132
Occupational therapists	£11
Home help	£104
Meals on Wheels	£18
General practitioner	£11
Drugs	£18
	£294 in 1972 prices

To estimate total costs it would then be necessary to estimate the
costs borne by the patient, his family, etc. However, even after
making allowance for such costs, it seems reasonable to accept Rickard's
conclusion that domiciliary care would be far cheaper than care in a
community hospital. Of course, this does not necessarily mean that
domiciliary care is superior since the benefits of treatment by the two
methods might be very different.

SUMMARY

The success of the community hospital policy will depend to a large
extent on the attitudes of doctors and other medical staff. In particular, community hospitals will need general practitioners to undertake
the day to day medical care of patients, consultants will have to be
willing to hold appropriate out-patient clinics in them and community
hospitals must be capable of attracting nurses, physiotherapists,
occupational therapists and radiographers to work in them.

Questionnaire surveys were conducted to find out the nature of local
medical opinion on the most appropriate functions of small local hospitals and the degree of enthusiasm and likely involvement of the relevant
Health Service staff groups. Hospital doctors were found to be

generally reluctant to release the in-patients at present under their care to peripheral units supervised by general practitioners. To accord with this viewpoint, community hospitals must for the most part provide beds to relieve the community rather than to relieve the general hospitals. Beds for this purpose were felt to be necessary by general practitioners. When asked to comment on the adequacy of various hospital services in the district, general practitioners identified as inadequate those services that the policy was expressly designed to improve. The implication of these findings is clearly for an increase in hospital beds in contradiction with the explicit Department of Health and Social Security policy that the provision of community hospitals should not add to the total number of hospital beds in a health district. In the long term it may be that the rehabilitative service community hospitals are intended to provide will tend to reduce the pressure on general hospital beds by extending the useful life of people in the community. In the short term however, the provision of community hospitals in rural districts such as the one studied appears certain to demand additional resources.

In general, both hospital doctors and general practitioners agreed with the DHSS guidelines for the functions of community hospitals. The one major exception was that the majority of doctors were not in favour of including the elderly mentally infirm and the nurses and rehabilitative staff members questioned were also notably unenthusiastic about working with this group of patients. It may be then, that fresh thought will be necessary on the policy of elderly persons with dementia. If our sample of hospital doctors is representative, it seems that generally consultants will agree to holding out-patient clinics in small local hospitals in those specialties where large numbers of patients may be seen without requiring the facilities of a district general hospital. We estimate that about 40% of out-patient attendances in the district studied fall into this category. Most general practitioners questioned indicated an interest in active participation, although it is notable that a large number of them volunteered the view that adequate remuneration would have to be provided and their existing workload would have to be reduced to make the scheme a success. For nurses and the other relevant groups of trained staff, the question is whether the distinctive size and character of a community hospital would be attractive as a workplace in the face of competition from district general hospitals. With the information available it seems that community hospitals will have rather more difficulty in attracting physiotherapists, occupational therapists and radiographers than nurses. This is disturbing as the function of the community hospital as a supportive and rehabilitative centre, particularly for day patients, is one of the cornerstones of the policy. The idea that community hospitals will be able to tap local pools of trained people not otherwise available to the Health Service is also shown by the evidence to be possibly over-optimistic.

The costs of caring for patients in community hospitals will have a vital influence on their feasibility and success. At present there is little firm evidence on this issue, but there are some indications that caring for patients in a community hospital might be cheaper than in a district general hospital and more expensive than domiciliary care. This does not suggest which of these alternatives is best since the different benefits from each would also need to be considered. There is also some evidence that for small local hospitals the minimum size above which average costs do not rise is about 35 beds, a figure somewhat below the 50 to 150 bed range suggested by the DHSS.

4 The costs to patients and visitors

When the relative merits of different hospital location strategies are debated, the health authority must consider the balance of the various costs involved. These costs may be divided into "internal" costs incurred by the health service itself and "external" or "social" costs, which are borne directly by the community. Both types of cost may be either monetary or non-monetary. Compared with internal costs, the costs to the community are difficult to assess and incorporate in the evaluative procedure. This chapter explores the expenditure and inconveniences of hospital patients and their visitors. Only the costs incurred by actual patients and their visitors are considered. That is, the social costs of not having the opportunity to be a hospital patient or to visit a hospital patient because the hospital services are inaccessible are ignored for the present. They will be the subject of the following chapter.

Of all the hospital service's costs that are borne by the community, those associated with travel are the ones obviously affected by hospital location policy. In rural areas, many residents have to travel long distances to attend out-patient clinics, to be admitted into hospital and to visit relatives and friends who are in hospital themselves. Such journeys can be time-consuming, costly and inconvenient. Furthermore, given the poor quality or even total absence of public transport in some places, transport problems are likely to be particularly difficult for those without the use of a car. People who are used to making the journey to a certain market town to reach their workplace, for shopping, schooling and entertainment, may discover that they must travel somewhere else for their local hospital. As well as the journey itself, there may be the difficulties of taking time off work or arranging for children to be looked after.

Before the costs to patients and visitors of any proposed planning strategies can be compared, information is needed on the situation at present: on the distances people typically travel to hospital in a rural area, the modes of transport they use, the time and monetary costs involved and the attendant inconveniences they experience.

THE QUESTIONNAIRE SURVEYS

In order to investigate some of the costs to the community associated with travel to hospital services in a rural area three questionnaire surveys were conducted. The first was a survey of out-patients attending clinics, the second was of non-psychiatric in-patients considered suitable for care in small local hospitals together with their visitors, and the third was of elderly mentally infirm hospital patients and their visitors. The organisation of the three surveys and the characteristics of the samples obtained will be described in turn.

Survey of out-patients

For a period of two weeks all out-patients attending certain clinics
in the West Norfolk and King's Lynn General Hospital, St. James'
Hospital, King's Lynn, and the North Cambridgeshire Hospital, Wisbech,
were given a questionnaire to complete by the clinic receptionist.
The questionnaire form is given in Appendix D.   Completed forms were
returned to the receptionist before the patient left the clinic.
In all, 53 clinic sessions were surveyed.   The specialties included
in the survey, in order of the number of sessions held during the
survey period, were: medicine, surgery, opthalmology, E.N.T.,
gynaecology, paediatrics, orthopaedics, geriatrics and rheumatology.
Altogether 722 forms were returned, of which 57% were at the King's
Lynn clinics and the remainder in Wisbech.   The out-patients in the
sample contained a preponderance of females (60%) and they varied in
age from under 15 to over 75 with the majority being in the middle of
this range (Table 4.1).   Most had been previously to the clinic but
for 26% that was their first attendance.

Table 4.1
Age of out-patients

Age	Number
Under 15	97
15-24	64
25-44	218
45-64	191
65-74	82
75+	35

Survey of preconvalescent and geriatric patients

The survey of non-psychiatric in-patients and their visitors was more
complicated as it involved a sampling procedure of several stages in
seven hospitals.   Four medical and surgical wards of the West Norfolk
and King's Lynn General Hospital, four orthopaedic and geriatric wards
of St. James' Hospital and the small chest and isolation unit,
Hardwick Hospital, were the places for the survey in the town of
King's Lynn.   In Wisbech, four medical and surgical wards of the
North Cambridgeshire Hospital and three geriatric and post operative
wards in the Clarkson Hospital were sampled.   The preconvalescent
unit at Stow Hall Hospital near Downham Market was included, as was
the 18-bed Swaffham Cottage Hospital, the only general practitioner
unit in the district.   Of the non-psychiatric, non-maternity hospitals
in the district only one (the Hunstanton Recovery Hospital for
convalescent patients) was omitted.

The survey consisted of an in-patient interview and a visitor
questionnaire.   The first step in the procedure was for a member of
the study team to visit the ward and request the Sister on duty to

identify any patients who were suitable to be looked after in a community hospital (defined as a small local hospital where nursing and rehabilitative care would be provided under the supervision of the patient's general practitioner). On the occasions when the Sister was absent, the staff nurse in charge was approached. It is impossible to say, of course, whether their judgements would have coincided with the opinions of consultants, but in cases of doubt the tendency was not to include the patient in the sample. Certainly in the general hospitals an extremely low proportion of patients (perhaps about 1% in the West Norfolk and King's Lynn General Hospital) were selected. Although this meant that only a small sample was identified, we are reasonably sure that unsuitable patients were effectively excluded.

The second stage was that those patients considered suitable for community hospital care who were not asleep or too ill to be disturbed were approached by the team member, who explained the survey and requested their permission to include them in it. A small proportion did not wish to be disturbed and were therefore not engaged any further. Others were too deaf to hear or appeared unable to understand and these people also were not included. The remaining patients, those who agreed to take part and who gave every sign of understanding, were interviewed to establish their length of stay, address, admission mode of transport, number of visitors, and so on. The form used by the interviewer appears as Appendix E. The patients were then given a small number of questionnaire forms for visitors (Appendix F) and asked to give them to their own visitors so that they could fill them in at the bedside and leave the completed forms with the patient. The interviewer let the patient know that she would return in two or three days to collect the forms. When the completed visitor questionnaire forms (if there were any) had been collected, the sampling procedure was complete. In many cases, no visitor forms were filled in, but the patient's questionnaire was still kept as part of the sample.

This procedure was followed in the seven hospitals for a total of eleven weeks, the interviewer returning to each ward when sufficient time had elapsed to produce a change of patients. The length of time necessary to accumulate a large enough sample emphasises a point made in the previous chapter : that "community hospital" patients are rarely to be found in the present acute hospital system. By the end of the period a sample of only 259 in-patients had been obtained. Completed questionnaires were received from 192 groups of visitors, consisting of 323 individual visitors. A high proportion of the patients (43%) yielded no completed visitor forms. A total of 109 patients returned one visitor form, 34 returned two forms and five patients returned three different visitor forms.

The number of in-patients interviewed in each of the hospitals ranged from only 10 in the West Norfolk and King's Lynn General Hospital to 88 in Stow Hall Hospital. As might be expected, it was the general practitioner hospital at Swaffham and Stow Hall pre-convalescent unit that yielded most in-patients for the survey relative to their bed numbers. That the largest and most specialised acute hospital produced the lowest number of "community hospital" patients was as expected. Of the 259 patients, only 40

were identified in geriatric wards.   The remaining 219 were in acute
wards.   This group of patients was termed "preconvalescent patients".
A minority, perhaps, were not strictly preconvalescent in the sense of
being patients who had already received the most intensive part of
their treatment but who still required active nursing care and medical
supervision.   The term was used for convenience, to distinguish the
non-geriatric medical and surgical patients considered suitable for a
community hospital from the 40 geriatric patients.

The ages and sex of the sample of in-patients are given in Table 4.2.
The sample contained a preponderance of female patients (57%) and also
of patients in the older age groups.   Also given in the table are the
national percentages of in-patients in each of the age/sex categories,
with which to compare the sample.   The national percentages do not
include psychiatric and maternity in-patients, nor do they include in-
patients less than 5 years old.

Table 4.2

Sample and national in-patients age and sex characteristics :
percentages

| Age | Males | | Females | |
(years)	Sample %	National %	Sample %	National %
5-14	1	6	0	5
15-44	10	13	8	21
45-64	13	14	19	13
65-74	11	8	13	7
75 and over	8	5	17	8
All ages	43	46	57	54

Source for national percentages : DHSS & OPCS (1974)

As the table demonstrates, the sex composition of the sample was
very close to what would be expected from the national in-patient
figures, the difference being only 3%.   In the younger groups the
sample contained proportionately less in-patients than those in the
national survey.   By contrast, the sample had proportionately more
patients over 65 years old than the national survey.   This bias
towards the elderly in the sample is entirely in keeping with the
observation that patients who do not need the specialised facilities
of a district general hospital but who nonetheless do need hospital
care tend to be the older rather than the younger in-patients.
Altogether 49% of the sample was over 65 years old, and 25% was over
75 years old.   While 71% of the male patients were married only
54% of the women were, the difference being accounted for by a higher
proportion of widowed and divorced women.

The age and sex characteristics of the visitors in the sample are
given in Table 4.3.   The table shows a spread over all age groups,
with a slight preponderance of female visitors over male visitors.

Table 4.3
Percentage age and sex distribution of visitors

Age	Male %	Female %
Under 15	3	4
15-24	5	5
25-44	15	20
45-64	13	18
65-74	5	8
75 and over	2	2
BASE	132	179

Slightly over half the visitors (52%) were the close relatives of the patient (either parents, sons, daughters, brothers, sisters, husbands or wives).   The remainder may be divided almost equally into less close relatives (25%) and friends and neighbours (21%). Fewer than 1.5% of the visitors in the sample were visiting as social workers or representatives of a voluntary body or church.

Visitor groups were defined as people who travelled to the hospital together.   A high proportion of groups (41%) consisted of a single visitor, 36% of groups were of two visitors and 15% consisted of three visitors.   Only 5% of groups had four members and 3% had five members.

Survey of elderly mentally infirm patients

The third questionnaire survey on the topic of costs to patients and visitors was a survey of elderly severely mentally infirm patients and their visitors.   As there are no hospital beds for this type of patient at present in the King's Lynn District it was necessary to conduct the survey outside the study area, in the neighbouring Norwich Health District.   The hospitals used were Hellesdon Hospital on the north-western outskirts of the city of Norwich and The Vale Hospital, Swainsthorpe, some five miles to the south of Norwich.   The patients in the sample included some from the King's Lynn District but also some from addresses nearer the hospitals, in the Norwich District. The procedure for the survey differed in several respects from that of the non-psychiatric in-patients survey.   Five psychogeriatric wards were selected in each hospital and in each ward the senior nurse with the most experience of the patients was requested to supply basic information about them.   Information on age, sex, marital status, home address and admission date was obtained for all patients and the senior nurses were also asked to estimate the number of different people visiting and the total number of visits in a typical month for each patient.   Ministers of the church and social workers were not included as visitors.   Visitor questionnaire forms identical to those used in the non-psychiatric in-patient survey (Appendix F) were left on the ward, to be handed by nurses to visitors when they arrived. Completed visitor forms were collected from the hospital one month later.

A total of 226 elderly mentally infirm patients were included in the study: 100 in Hellesdon Hospital and 126 in The Vale Hospital. The majority (75%) were female and 73% of them were aged 75 and over. 32% of the men and 19% of the women had spouses still living.

Although the survey period extended over one month, visitor forms were completed by only 90 groups, consisting of 162 people. The sizes of groups were similar to those in the non-psychiatric in-patient survey, but this time the most popular group size was two persons (37%), followed by one person (32%), three people (20%), four (10%) and five people (1%). Close relatives of the patient made up 62% of the recorded visitors, a higher proportion than in the non-psychiatric survey. Other relatives accounted for about 20% and friends and neighbours for 17%. Again, the majority of visitors were female, but the ages of visitors to elderly mentally infirm patients (Table 4.4) were higher than those recorded in the previous survey, as might be expected.

Table 4.4

Percentage age and sex distribution of visitors to elderly mentally infirm patients

Age	Male %	Female %
Under 15	1	1
15-24	3	2
25-44	21	17
45-64	50	52
65-74	14	16
75 and over	11	12
BASE	66	87

THE JOURNEY TO HOSPITAL

The difficulties patients and visitors experience in going to hospital depend to some extent on circumstances such as having to take time off work, to make special arrangements for children or to ask a friend to be a companion on the trip, but the most basic factors that determine how easy it is to get to hospital are the distance involved and the mode of transport used. The patients and visitors included in the surveys were asked questions on where they lived, where they started their journey to hospital and how they travelled. The exception was in the case of the elderly mentally infirm patients, for whom no transport information was sought as most had been originally admitted some years previously, often to a different hospital. Information was available for out-patients, preconvalescent and geriatric in-patients and for the visitors to both this group of in-patients and the elderly mentally infirm group. It will be presented in that order.

Journeys of out-patients

Out-patient clinics are at present held only in the larger hospitals and this limited the journeys made by out-patients in the sample to two destinations: King's Lynn and Wisbech. Table 4.5 shows the distribution of straight line distances out-patients travelled to their clinics. Many out-patients travelled from within King's Lynn or Wisbech and therefore had journeys of less than two miles. Only a fifth of the total had journeys longer than ten miles and considerably less than one percent travelled more than 20 miles. Some of the journeys from within the two towns, however, were made by people who lived elsewhere, but visited the clinic from work. In the majority of cases (86%) the trip to the clinic started from the patient's home but 11% of respondents came to the clinic from work and the remaining few from other origins. Of the trips which started from work approximately 70% were from within King's Lynn or Wisbech. Whatever the origin of their trip, an overwhelming majority of people (96%) came straight from there to the clinic. After leaving the clinic most people (72%) intended to return home; on the return journey a higher proportion than on the outward journey were going to work (14%) or to another destination (13%). It therefore seems that a substantial minority of out-patient trips are not simple home-based ones.

Table 4.5
Out-patients' distance travelled to clinic

Distance	% Out-patients
0-2 miles	42
2-10 miles	38
10-20 miles	20
Over 20 miles	0
BASE	722

The King's Lynn District has already been identified as a district with particularly high car ownership levels and this was borne out by the sample of out-patients. Only 22% of the out-patients were from households that did not own a car. One car households were the most frequent category encountered (65% of the sample) but two and and three car households accounted for 11% and 2% of the sample respectively. Over half (52%) of the out-patients questioned possessed a driving licence. A high proportion, therefore, might be expected to travel by private car to the clinic. Table 4.6 confirms that a majority of the respondents did indeed use private cars for their journey to the out-patient clinic. Many of them drove themselves but a larger number had to be driven, often by someone outside their own household. This being the case, many trips to out-patient clinics consumed the time not only of the patient but also of a driver. Of those given a lift in a non household car, only 13% made a contribution towards the costs of the journey.

Table 4.6
Out-patients' mode of transport

Mode	%
Ambulance	2
Hospital car service	9
Household car (driver)	30
Household car (passenger)	22
Non-household car (passenger)	11
Foot/bicycle	14
Bus/train	10
Taxi	1
Other	1

The other significant modes were the hospital car service, public transport by bus or train and by bicycle or on foot. Each of these accounted for a considerable number of people but in all cases substantially fewer than the private car. Other modes were relatively unimportant in terms of the numbers using them. It is worth noting that the mode was the same in both directions for 95% of trips.

Although Table 4.6 shows the modes of transport used for the whole of the sample it is likely that the importance of different modes will not be the same for all groups. Because women less often have access to a car and are less often able to drive, fewer women than men might use a private car to get to an out-patient clinic. Similarly, there might be differences between car owning and non car owning households and between people of different ages. The length of the journey could also affect the mode of transport used.

Table 4.7 shows that a higher proportion of men than women came as car drivers whereas women were more likely to be car passengers. Considering together the figures for car drivers and passengers a slightly higher proportion of men came by private car. Correspondingly, a higher proportion of women used the hospital car service or public transport.

Table 4.7
Out-patients' mode of transport by sex

Mode	Males %	Females %
Hospital car service	7	10
Ambulance	2	3
Household car (driver)	38	25
Household car (passenger)	28	38
Foot/bicycle	14	13
Bus/train	8	11
Other	3	1

This pattern is repeated in a more marked form when car-owning and non car owning households are compared. Out-patients from non car owning households were much less likely to use a private car for the journey to the clinic but still almost a quarter of them travelled by private car (Table 4.8).

Table 4.8
Out-patients' mode of transport by car ownership

Mode	Car Owning %	Non Car Owning %
Hospital car service	4	24
Ambulance	2	5
Car (driver)	38	0
Car (passenger)	37	23
Foot/bicycle	9	29
Bus/train	8	16
Other	2	2

The relationship between the mode of transport used and the age of the respondent was much less marked. The most noteworthy feature was that the use of the private car decreased steadily with age beyond the 25-44 years age group, where the proportion was 70%. For the 45-64 years group the proportion was 62%, which declined to 59% and 51% for those out-patients aged 65-74 and over 75 respectively. Rather surprisingly, the proportion of out-patients using public transport remained steady at ten or eleven percent for all age groups.

One further issue which was investigated was whether those coming relatively long distances to the out-patient clinics used different modes of transport than those with shorter journeys. Certain differences are fairly obvious. For example, walking and cycling was a significant mode of transport only within the towns of King's Lynn and Wisbech (Table 4.9). By contrast, the use of health service transport increased with distance, particularly for those from non car owning households. This mode was used more by those people in the remoter parts of the district, many of which have poor public transport. Rather more surprising was the relationship between public transport use and distance. For car owning households the use of public transport was greater for the longer trips than for the shorter ones. This trend is the reverse of the trend of public transport quality. For the shorter journeys the frequency of buses will tend to be greater, the costs will be lower and journey times will be less. That is, one might expect public transport to be a more attractive mode for short rather than long journeys. In spite of the disadvantages of public transport for long journeys it seems that it was more often used for this type of journey. The use of private cars was considerably less for trips of over 10 miles than for those of 2-10 miles, even though the car might be the most convenient mode of transport for relatively long journeys in rural areas. A possible reason for this pattern of behaviour in car owning households is that the car may not be easily released from its journey to work function for people who live in remote places. Whatever the reason, the situation revealed by the survey was that many people travelling long distances to out-patient clinics not only faced the difficulties posed by these long distances, but also were subject to the additional problems of using public transport.

Table 4.9
Out-patients' transport mode by distance and car ownership

Car Ownership:	Car Owning			Non Car Owning		
Distance (miles)	0-2	2-10	10+	0-2	2-10	10+
	%	%	%	%	%	%
Ambulance/hospital car	3	6	11	14	32	59
Car	68	87	74	24	32	18
Bus/train	5	7	15	7	33	23
Foot/bicycle	24	0	0	55	3	0

Journeys of preconvalescent and geriatric in-patients

This group of in-patients had travelled not only to hospitals in King's Lynn and Wisbech but also to the units at Swaffham and Downham Market. Information on the distribution of their homes is of interest because it is evidence (albeit limited evidence from a small sample) of the catchments of the hospitals. From an examination of the distances between in-patients' homes and various hospitals it ought to be possible to judge to what extent each hospital in the study area is serving its immediate locality and to what extent it is being used as a district hospital. The straight line distances between in-patients' homes and the hospital in which they were interviewed are given in Table 4.10 which shows considerable differences between the four hospital towns. The evidence of the sample is that the hospitals in Wisbech and Swaffham draw on a very restricted catchment area. In a sense, then, hospitals in these two towns are acting as local "community" hospitals already. In Wisbech hospitals 91% of the sample of patients lived within 10 miles, and the corresponding figure was 97% for Swaffham. The very different function of Stow Hall Hospital near Downham Market is reflected in its figures. Only 23% of the sample there lived within 10 miles, the remaining 77% living further than 10 miles away. The King's Lynn hospitals fall between these extremes, with 41% of patients in the sample from within 10 miles. In contrast to those at Wisbech and Swaffham, hospitals in King's Lynn and Downham have a "district" catchment area which Downham is less able to serve efficiently as it lies further away from the main centres of population.

Table 4.10
Distance between in-patients' homes and hospital, by hospital
location

Distance	King's Lynn %	Wisbech %	Downham %	Swaffham %
0-2 miles	23	35	7	39
2-10 miles	18	56	16	58
10-20 miles	49	4	59	3
Over 20 miles	10	5	18	0
BASE	68	72	88	31

Table 4.11 shows the replies of in-patients to the question "How
did you get to hospital when you were first admitted?", broken down
by the home to hospital distance.   Altogether almost three quarters
of patients travelled by ambulance but it is possible that this figure
is higher than that applying to original admissions to hospital since
a proportion of patients in the sample had been transferred (by
ambulance) from another hospital to the unit in which they were interviewed.   Approximately 22% of the patients had not used Health Service
transport to get to hospital and of these the overwhelming majority
travelled by car.   About 8% of the whole sample had accepted a lift in
a car not belonging to their own household and none of these poeple had
contributed towards the cost of the journey, which had therefore been
borne by "outsiders".   The table shows that public transport is of
negligible importance for in-patient admission, although it was used
more for longer journeys than for shorter journeys.   As in the out-
patient survey, noticeably lower proportions of patients travelled by
car for distances greater than ten miles than for lesser distances.
The gap this creates is principally filled by the ambulance service.

Table 4.11
Transport mode used for admission, by distance

Mode	0-2 miles %	2-10 miles %	Over 10 miles %
Ambulance	63	59	86
Hospital car service	7	8	2
Household car (driver)	2	1	1
Household car (passenger)	16	15	4.5
Non-household car (passenger)	5	15	4.5
Foot or bicycle	5	1	0
Bus or train	0	1	2
Taxi	2	0	0
BASE	58	81	111

Visiting journeys to preconvalescent and geriatric in-patients

The distances travelled by visitors to reach the hospitals in the four towns are given in Table 4.12. A marked difference is apparent between the towns. While a very high proportion of visitors to hospitals in Wisbech and Swaffham come from less than ten miles away (85% and 84% respectively), the corresponding figures for King's Lynn and Downham Market are much lower (47% for King's Lynn and a mere 21% for Downham). With 79% of its visitors travelling more than 10 miles, the hospital at Downham Market is particularly remote.

Table 4.12
Distances travelled by visiting groups, by hospital location

Distance	King's Lynn %	Wisbech %	Downham %	Swaffham %
0-2 miles	23	34	5	39
2-10 miles	24	51	16	45
10-20 miles	41	7	60	10
Over 20 miles	12	8	19	6
BASE	34	59	68	31

Table 4.12 closely resembles Table 4.10, which showed the distribution of in-patient home distances from hospital. The resemblance is no coincidence, of course, for visitors tend to live in the same places as the patients they come to visit. It is useful to explore the connection between patients' homes and their visitors' homes. If a strong connection exists it would be possible to make an estimate of the origins of visitors from the home locations of patients. The distribution of distances between the homes of the patients in the sample and the homes of the people who visit them in hospital appear in Table 4.13. Fully two thirds of the visitors to hospital lived within two miles of the patients they went to visit. The remaining third lived in a wide range of distances from their respective in-patients' homes, but with a preponderance in the 2-10 miles category.

The significance of Table 4.13 is that it allows predictions to be made. When assessing different hospital locations it would be useful if their implications in terms of visitors' travelling distances could be measured. This has not been done up to now because there has been no method to estimate where the visitors are likely to come from. Once the origins of in-patients are determined, however, Table 4.13 can be used to allocate potential visitors around each in-patient. Two thirds of the visitors lived in the same parish or town as the patient they wished to visit and further analysis showed that the proportion did not vary significantly with distance to the hospital. The geographical origins of the majority of visitors may therefore be estimated using this result. Allocating the remaining third over the Health District could be achieved by designating concentric probability zones around each in-patient location, but a much simpler method would be to spread them over the district in proportion to the population of each parish or town.

Table 4.13
Distances from patients' home to their visitors' homes

Distance	%
0-2 miles	67
2-10 miles	20
10-20 miles	5
Over 20 miles (within Health District)	5
Over 20 miles (outside Health District)	3
BASE	188

The majority of visitors began their journey to the hospital at home and returned home after the visit. Altogether 15% of journeys did not follow this pattern (Table 4.14). To measure visiting distances from the home to the hospital therefore involves a small amount of error. Since workplaces and "other" origins and destinations (for example visits to friends, shopping, etc) will tend to be in the larger centres where the hospitals are also situated, the number of short distance journeys will tend to be slightly underestimated and the number of longer journeys to be slightly overestimated by home to hospital distances.

Table 4.14
Origins and destinations of visitor groups

Destinations:	% of all trips		
	Home	Work	Other
Origins: Home	85	1	4
Work	2	3	0
Other	3	0	3

Visitors were asked to indicate their mode of transport to the hospital and they were also asked whether they intended to leave in the same manner. As with the out-patients, changes in mode proved to be very rare: over 98% of groups intended to use the same mode of transport in their journey away from the hospital. The frequencies of modes used are given in Table 4.15. The large majority travelled "under their own steam" (by car, motorcycle, bicycle or on foot). In this category were 93% of the groups, compared with less than 6% relying upon public transport and taxis.

By far the most popular mode was the car, used by 78% of groups. Of the visitors who travelled by car, exactly half were the drivers, 35% were passengers in their own household car and 14% were passengers in another car (1% was recorded as "none of these"). The ratios were not greatly affected by age: of the people aged 65-74 who travelled by car, 40% drove the vehicle, and this was reduced only to 33% in the over 75 age group. The second most popular mode (walking and cycling) was a long way behind the car in terms of frequency of use and, as will be seen later, it was a significant mode only for short distances. Only ten groups (5% of the sample) travelled by public transport, and four of these were from within King's Lynn and Wisbech. Of the remaining six, four were from parishes with "good" public transport (more than 15 buses per day, Monday to Friday) and two were from parishes with "intermediate" public transport (1-15 buses per day, Monday to Friday). None came from villages with a poorer service. Thus the few visiting groups who did use public transport came from parishes with comparatively good bus services.

Table 4.15
Visitors' mode of transport

	Groups %	Individuals %
Car	78	85
Motorcycle	1	0.5
Foot/bicycle	14	10
Bus/train	5	3
Taxi	0.5	0.5
Other	1	1
BASE	191	316

As well as the distribution of groups according to transport mode, Table 4.15 also gives the mode of transport of individual visitors. Because groups travelling by car tended to be larger than groups travelling by bus, the percentage of individuals using a car (85%) was even higher than the corresponding percentage for groups and, similarly, the proportion travelling by bus was reduced to a mere 3% when individuals rather than groups were considered. Thus, measured in terms of the number of people involved, only an insignificant proportion of visitors travelled by public transport or taxi. The conclusion must be that in circumstances where travel by car, foot or bicycle is not possible some potential visiting trips are not made.

Table 4.16 illustrates that car users, bus and train passengers and those who walk or cycle all had their own characteristic distribution of group sizes. Car users travelled in groups of from one to five people, their most popular group size being two people. Only 30% of car users visited the hospital alone, while about 80% of both bus passengers and walkers came on their own. This difference may be partly a reflection of the fact that doubling the number of visitors doubles the cost or effort for bus passengers and walkers, whereas the same is not true for car users, but it may also stem from the differences in household composition between users of the different modes (for example, single person households are less likely to own a car).

Although the numbers are small and not reliable, they suggest that bus travel inhibits larger groups of visitors to a greater extent than walking.

Table 4.16
Group size of visitors by mode of transport

Group size	Car %	Foot/bicycle %	Bus/train %
1 person	30	78	80
2 people	43	7	20
3 people	17	11	-
4 people	7	-	-
5 people	3	4	-
BASE	149	27	10

Not surprisingly, the mode of transport used by a group of visitors was strongly related to the length of the journey (Table 4.17). For distances of less than two miles almost as many people walked or cycled as made the trip by car. As the distance increased from two miles, there was a sudden decrease in the percentage of groups walking and cycling and a corresponding increase in the car and bus journeys. Even so, the proportion of groups travelling by bus did not exceed 8% at any distance, while the proportion of car users fluctuated at a high level, around 90%.

Table 4.17
Visitor groups' mode of transport by distance travelled

	0-2 miles %	2-10 miles %	10-20 miles %	Over 20 miles %
Car	51	87	86	93
Foot or bicycle	47	6	2	-
Bus or train	2	5	8	7
Other	-	2	4	-
BASE	43	62	61	15

Visiting journeys to the elderly mentally infirm

As was mentioned earlier, there is no hospital provision for the elderly mentally infirm in the King's Lynn District so it was necessary to collect information on visiting trips to these patients in two hospitals, one on the outskirts of Norwich and one near the village of Swainsthorpe, Norfolk. Since these hospitals draw on an extensive

area which includes the King's Lynn District as well as the Norwich
District it is expected that the distances travelled by visitors must
considerably exceed those of the hospital visitors just described.
The origins of the sample of patients in the two psychiatric hospitals
are indicated by Table 4.18, in which the high proportion of patients
whose homes were more than 20 miles distant is noteworthy. The "bulge"
in the second distance category for the hospital at Swainsthorpe is due
to its admissions from Norwich.

Table 4.18
Distance between elderly mentally infirm patients' homes and
hospital, by hospital location

Distance	Norwich %	Swainsthorpe %
0-2 miles	34	2
2-10 miles	10	53
10-20 miles	14	20
Over 20 miles	41	25
BASE	97	118

The distribution of distances travelled by visitors to these patients
is given in Table 4.19. While about one fifth of visitors did travel
more than 20 miles, the proportions in the higher distance categories
are perhaps not as large as might have been anticipated from Table 4.18.
Whether the survey produced evidence of trip suppression with increasing distance will be discussed in Chapter 5.

Table 4.19
Distances travelled by visiting groups to elderly mentally infirm
patients, by hospital location

Distance	Norwich %	Swainsthorpe %
0-2 miles	27	5
2-10 miles	29	56
10-20 miles	23	19
Over 20 miles	21	19
BASE	48	41

As with the visitors to non-psychiatric patients, a majority lived
within two miles of the patients' home, but for this group the proportion was lower, at 56%. Altogether 25% of visitors lived within
2-10 miles of the patient's home, 8% within 10-20 miles and 11% over
20 miles away. Even more of the visitors to elderly mentally infirm
patients started and finished their journey at home (Table 4.20)

compared with the visiting trips to preconvalescent and geriatric patients.

Table 4.20

Origins and destinations of visitor groups to elderly mentally infirm patients

Destinations:	% of all trips		
	Home	Work	Other
Origins: Home	90	1	3
Work	2	0	0
Other	4	0	0

Again, by far the most frequent mode of transport was the car, used by 86% of groups. Public transport was much more popular than with the first sample of visitors and accounted for 12% of group trips. The remaining 2% of groups were evenly divided between walking or cycling and travelling by taxi. The reason for the greater popularity of public transport compared with the first survey of visitors is not clear, but it may stem from the greater proportion of elderly people in the sample of visitors to elderly mentally infirm patients and also from the regular suburban bus service linking Hellesdon Hospital to the centre of Norwich. The hospital at Swainsthorpe has a once-weekly bus service to the door from central Norwich which, as will be seen when visiting rates are described in the next chapter, is not too infrequent for most visitors.

TRAVEL TIME AND COST

In the survey of out-patients and the two surveys of visitors to hospital, respondents were asked about the length of time their journeys had taken and those travelling by public transport were asked to state the single fare. Their replies were used to establish the range of travel times and costs to be expected in a rural health district, to compare the differences between private and public transport users and to investigate the relationship between the time taken and the distance travelled.

Time and distance

The frequency distribution of travel times for the sample of out-patients is given in Table 4.21. The time taken to reach the clinic was relatively short for most people. About a third of the respondents took ten minutes or less whilst 86% were able to reach the clinic in 30 minutes or less. Given the rural nature of the district, this seems a not unsatisfactory state of affairs for the majority (although we do not know how many potential out-patients were not referred to the clinic because of the long journey time). Of the remaining 14% who took longer than half an hour a small proportion did report journeys exceeding one hour.

98

Table 4.21
Time taken for trip to out-patient clinic

Time	% Out-patients
0-10 minutes	35
11-20 minutes	29
21-30 minutes	22
31-60 minutes	13
1 - 2 hours	1
BASE	702

Rather longer times were needed to get to the hospital by both samples of visitors (Table 4.22). A majority of them travelled to the hospital in less than half an hour, but it was a smaller majority than that of the out-patients sample. The proportion of visitors taking longer than one hour was also appreciably higher, especially in the case of visitors to the elderly mentally infirm who, it will be recalled, were more likely to be elderly themselves and to travel by bus. It may well be that some of the "slower" visitors would be of the type to receive health service transport if they were out-patients. This may help to explain the difference between Tables 4.21 and 4.22. Of the visitors whose journey time exceeded two hours, in the preconvalescent sample all had travelled from outside the district and in the elderly mentally infirm sample two out of five groups were from outside the district.

Table 4.22
Visitors' travel times to hospital

Time	Preconvalescent and geriatric sample %	Elderly mentally infirm sample %
0-30 minutes	79	62
31-60 minutes	16	23
1 - 2 hours	4	9
Over 2 hours	1	6
BASE	184	88

The time taken on the journey to hospital is a function of the mode of transport and the distance. Statistical analysis of the out-patients sample, which is the largest sample of the three surveys, can be used to measure the average speed by car, bus or health service transport. Table 4.23 shows the result of fitting linear regression equations to the data which were disaggregated by transport mode and destination. The regression equations express the average relationship between the journey time and the straight line distance measured on the map from the parish of origin to the hospital.

Table 4.23
Relationships between journey time, mode and distance

Mode	Regression Equation	Correlation coefficient	Number in sample
Car	T = 6.75 + 2.10D	0.80	434
Bus	T = 13.63 + 2.86D	0.77	67
Hospital transport	T = 10.20 + 1.99D	0.80	68

Note :   T = time in minutes: D = straight line distance in miles

For car users, the time includes not only the car travelling time but also the time involved in town traffic delays, parking, walking from the car to the clinic and also perhaps in finding the clinic.   The constant 6.75 is the average number of minutes spent at this stage of the trip by car users.   This time was taken on average whether the trip was a long or a short one and was additional to the actual driving time.   The constant 2.10 was the average number of minutes per mile. Translated into a more familiar miles per hour figure, the average speed was 28.6 mph.   This speed refers to the straight line map distances between places, which were used throughout this study as they could easily be measured by computer from information about the map coordinates of parishes and hospitals.   As the ratio between road distances and straight distances is known to be remarkably steady in most areas, subsequent conversion from one to the other can be readily achieved.   Analysis of straight and road distances from the 157 parishes and towns of the study district to the centre of King's Lynn established that road distances on the average were 1.15 times longer than straight distances.   The correlation between the two types of distance measure was very high (r = 0.97), so conversion could safely be made with little error.   After applying the correction factor, the average car speed on the road was found to be approximately 33 mph.

For bus travellers, the constant 13.63 was the average time incurred independently of journey distance.   This time included getting to the bus stop, waiting for the bus, being delayed by town traffic and walking from the destination stop to the clinic.   The average number of minutes taken by bus users to travel one straight line mile was 2.86 which, when the correction is applied, gives an average road speed of 24 mph.

Out-patients who were taken to the clinic by ambulance or hospital car had an average waiting time of 10.2 minutes, irrespective of the length of their journey.   Their average of 1.99 minutes per straight mile gave them an average road speed of almost 35 mph, which was slightly faster than private car users and considerably faster than the bus travellers.

The average time differences between the different modes of transport may be illustrated by applying the regression equations.   A five mile journey as the crow flies would take an average of 17 minutes by car, 28 minutes by bus and 20 minutes by ambulance or hospital car.   A ten mile journey (measured in a straight line) would take an average of 28 minutes by car, 42 minutes by bus and 30 minutes by health service transport.

Although the regression equations express the average relationship
between time and distance, by no means all the trips came close to
the average. This is shown by the correlation coefficients, which all
indicate a moderately strong association between time and distance, but
not a perfect relationship which would make the time of any particular
trip predictable from its distance. The variability of individual
journeys can be illustrated by referring to two examples from the
visitors to preconvalescent patients survey. One bus journey within
the town of King's Lynn was reported as having taken 45 minutes
altogether and another from two miles outside Downham Market to the
nearby Stow Hall Hospital took an hour. These are extreme cases, but
it is important to recognise that extreme cases do exist and that they
are ignored when predictions from average relationships are made.

For the out-patients who walked to the clinic, only a weak relationship between time and distance emerged. The journeys of walkers took
an average of 34 minutes. Once again, the actual walking times recorded were very variable around this average.

Cost

The surveys collected data on the costs of journeys only for those
respondents who travelled by public transport. For these people, costs
will clearly be related to the distances travelled, and, since the
distance travelled by public transport varied considerably, there are
likely to be wide variations in the amounts paid. Table 4.24 confirms
this for the sample of out-patients, showing that the cost of the single
fare to the clinic ranged from under 20 pence to over 80 pence, with
most people paying 60 pence or less (that is, less than £1.20 for the
return trip). This suggests that costs were low for the majority, but
for a minority they were more substantial. Of course, if the patient
was accompanied by someone else, the cost would be multiplied.

Table 4.24
Cost of single public transport trip to out-patients clinics

Cost	% Out-patients
0-20p	35
21-40p	23
41-60p	32
61-80p	4
81p or more	6
BASE	69

The surveys of visitors found only 21 groups travelling by public
transport in total, so only limited observations may be made about their
costs.   For eleven of the groups the single fare was less than 50p, so
that the return fare was less than £1.   The remainder (almost half)
paid more than 50p for the outward journey.   Three groups travelling
from outside the district reported single fares in the range £3 to £6.
Costs of this size when they do occur must act as a considerable
deterrent to people who have no access to a car and whose relative or
friend is admitted to a distant or inaccessible hospital.   Additionally, the more modest costs incurred by most visitors may become
burdensome when they are frequently repeated over a long period.   Of
course we have no measure of the number of potential visitors who were
deterred by the cost, only of those who were not deterred despite the
cost.

The average relationship between public transport cost and distance
was found by applying regression analysis to the cost and distance
information for the out-patients who travelled from within the district.
A linear regression equation was found to fit the data just as well as
a non-linear one, with a correlation coefficient of 0.7.   The
equation was:

$$C = 11.37 + 3.31 D \qquad (4.1)$$

where C was the cost of the single journey in pence and D was the
straight line distance in miles.   According to this equation, the
average amount paid for a single journey by an out-patient was 28p for
5 miles, 44p for 10 miles and 61p for 15 miles.   Outside this range
(that is, at distances greater than 15 miles) there were very few
observations and it may be that the equation slightly overestimates the
fare for longer distances because the actual cost per mile tends to
fall with increasing distance.   For the range of out-patient trips
encountered in the King's Lynn District, however, the equation allows
cost to be estimated if the distance of the journey is known.

Although the surveys asked no questions about the travel costs of
those who travelled to clinics by modes other than public transport,
in most such cases costs would have been incurred.   These may have
been paid by the patient, by somebody else or by the health service if
health service transport was used.   The difficulties of measuring
ambulance and hospital car service costs per mile have already been
discussed in Chapter 2;   here it is sufficient to recall that they are
high by comparison with other modes.   For the majority of out-patients
and visitors to hospital who travel by car, costs may be estimated
from the average running costs of a vehicle.   Since the need to visit
hospital is unlikely to determine whether or not a car is acquired
(except in the most extreme cases) the fixed costs such as those for a
car licence, insurance, depreciation and so on should not be included
in the calculation.   The relevant costs are the running costs, which
are directly dependent upon mileage.   Petrol accounts for about half
the running costs of an average vehicle and the remainder is accounted
for by oil, tyres, servicing and repairs.   For an average car with an
engine capacity of 1,000 to 1,500 cc the running cost in 1977 was 5.755
pence per mile (Automobile Association Technical Services, 1977).
This figure refers to road distances; the equivalent value for straight
line distances is 6.618 pence per mile.   Thus, a journey to a hospital
ten miles away on the map by car would cost about 66 pence and the

return trip would cost about £1.32.   The cost would almost certainly
seem to be lower than this to most car users, for whom the cost of
petrol is the most obvious measure of journey cost.

INCONVENIENCES OF THE HOSPITAL TRIP

While the difficulties of the trip to hospital are largely made up of
the time and cost involved, other costs (not necessarily monetary ones)
may be more important in some cases.   Working people who cannot easily
take time off and mothers with young children, for example, are expected to experience difficulties in addition to the simple journey costs.
On the other hand, simple journey time and cost information neglects
the fringe benefits a trip to the hospital might bring.   If the
hospital trip is combined with a shopping trip, for example, then the
journey cost should not be ascribed to the hospital visit alone.   A
special journey to a strange place is much less convenient that the
same length of journey frequently undertaken for other purposes.
To explore these hidden benefits and inconveniences of the hospital
trip we again refer to the surveys of out-patients and visitors.

Out-patients' special arrangements

A visit to a hospital clinic could necessitate a variety of special
arrangements.   It might be necessary to arrange transport, for example,
or for someone to accompany the out-patient.   Additionally, the visit
to the clinic might require that special arrangements be made at home
or at work.   The survey collected information on each of these aspects.

   Analysis of the modes of transport used to travel to out-patient
clinics showed that many people travelled as car passengers.   For two-
thirds of these people this involved being driven in the household car,
but the remaining third had to arrange transport in a car owned by a
relative, friend or neighbour.   No doubt in some cases this was not
easy.

   Many of the out-patients were accompanied on their visit to the
clinic (Table 4.25).   Most of those were accompanied by one person but
as many as 17% were accompanied by 2 or more people.   For the majority
of out-patients, then, the visit to a clinic involves the time and in
some cases the monetary costs incurred by companions.   Furthermore,
out-patients travelling longer distances were more likely to be
accompanied.   For distances of 0-2 miles, 46% of out-patients were
accompanied, compared with 61% and 59% for distances of 2-10 miles and
over 10 miles respectively.   The tendency of accompanied journeys to
be the longer ones is expected to raise costs significantly.

Table 4.25
People accompanying out-patient

Number of companions	% Out-patients
Nobody	44
1 person	39
2 people	11
3 or more people	6

Table 4.26 shows what special arrangements had to be made at home or work because of the trip to a clinic. Some of these are specific to particular types of people. Obviously, only those who work might have to take time off work and only those with children might have to make special arrangements for them to be looked after. Unfortunately no information was collected on the number of people who worked or had young children and therefore it is impossible, for example, to say what proportion of people who work had to take time off. However, the fact that a substantial proportion of those interviewed said that they had to make special arrangements of one kind or another suggests that the need to do this is widespread.

Table 4.26
Special arrangements made by out-patients

Arrangements	% Out-patients
For children	9
Time off work (unpaid)	10
Time off work (paid)	15
Someone else off work (accompanying patient)	6
Someone else off work (stays home)	1
Other	5

The most common special arrangement that had to be made was that the out-patient had to take time off work. Of those who had to do this 40% lost pay. For these people the trip to the clinic involved financial costs over and above the costs of the journey. Clearly, for them the accessibility of the clinic from their place of work is of greater importance than its accessibility from their home. A rather smaller number of respondents said that someone else had had to take time off work because of their trip to the clinic. In most cases this was so that they could accompany the patient. The other notable special arrangement was that some out-patients had to ask somebody to look after their children whilst they were away.

The question arises to what extent these special arrangements were dependent upon the distance to the clinic and therefore to what extent they might be reduced if hospitals were nearer. Of the out-patients who travelled less than two miles, 40% said they had to make special arrangements. The corresponding figures for those travelling 2-10 miles was 43% and 45% for journeys over 10 miles. The apparent slight increase was not statistically significant at the 0.05 level. This suggests that even if out-patients clinics were relocated to be nearer the people who currently face long journeys, this would not significantly reduce their need to make the special arrangements listed in Table 4.26, although it would reduce the length of time involved.

Multi-purpose trips

The surveys of out-patients and hospital visitors investigated the extent to which people also undertook other activities near the hospital. Where they were able to combine other activities with the trip to the hospital it seems reasonable to conclude that they were able to derive greater benefits from the trip than they would have done from a journey solely to the hospital. These additional benefits would offset some of the time and money costs of the trip. In some cases, of course, the additional activities might represent little more than "killing time" and hence their benefits to the patient might be small.

Of the sample of out-patients, 55% did nothing other than make the trip between home and the clinic. Amongst the 45% who mixed other activities with their trip the main activities were shopping and work (Table 4.27). However, only 30% said they would have needed to come to town anyway. From this it seems that about 15% of the out-patients would not otherwise have visited King's Lynn or Wisbech on that day and were using the trip to the clinic as an opportunity for shopping and a range of other activities.

Table 4.27
Other activities in town during day of visit to out-patient clinic

Activity	% Out-patients
Shopping	20
Children to or from school	6
Go to work	14
Go to bank	4
Go to post office	3
Other	6

The extent to which the clinic visit was mixed with other activities was not found to be the same for all groups. There were statistically significant tendencies (measured by a chi-square test at the 0.05 level) for higher proportions of certain groups to undertake additional activities during their trip. The proportions undertaking additional activities tended to be greater for people from car owning households, for those with a current driving licence, for younger adults and for those living relatively close to the out-patient clinic. It therefore appears that, as might be expected, the more mobile groups and those more accessible to the main towns are more likely to undertake other activities in King's Lynn or Wisbech during the day of their visit to the clinic. Those for whom the trip to the out-patient clinic is likely to be most difficult - the less mobile and those living furthest from the main towns - are less likely to undertake other activities in the town during the day of their visit.

For the two samples of visitors, people who lived in the same town as the hospital they were visiting were excluded from the analysis. The additional activities of visitor groups are shown against the towns they were visiting in Table 4.28. Again shopping and work were the only significant additional activities. Visitors were more likely to be shoppers and local workers in Wisbech and Swaffham than in King's Lynn and Norwich, and by a large margin, Downham Market and Swainsthorpe. Perhaps this is related to the distance of the hospital to the town centre, which is least in the case of Wisbech and Swaffham, but it must also be a function of the size of the hospitals' admissions catchment areas and the facilities of the towns. Conveying children to and from school, going to the bank and visiting the post office were activities of only a small minority of visitors.

Table 4.28
Other activities in conjunction with the visiting trip, by hospital town

Activity	Preconvalescent and geriatric patients				E.M.I. patients	
	King's Lynn	Wisbech	Downham	Swaffham	Norwich	Swains- thorpe
	%	%	%	%	%	%
Shopping	15	18	2	21	10	2
School	0	3	0	0	0	0
Work	8	18	5	16	8	7
Bank	0	0	0	0	2	0
Post Office	0	3	0	0	0	0
Other	0	11	5	11	2	2
BASE	26	38	62	19	48	41

E.M.I. = elderly mentally infirm

Comparison of the three samples of groups travelling to hospital showed a decreasing likelihood of taking advantage of the trip for other activities, from the out-patients (with the highest likelihood) through the preconvalescent patients' visitors to the visitors to elderly mentally infirm patients, who had the lowest likelihood. To illustrate, for shopping the proportions were: 20%, 11% and 7%. For work, the figures were: 14%, 10% and 8%; and for any other reported activity: 19%, 8% and 3%. This trend cannot be assumed to exist outside the study area, however, because it is complicated by the effect of the different hospital locations.

When asked whether they would have needed to visit the town anyway, 13% of groups coming to visit preconvalescent patients from outside the town replied "Yes" and 87% "No". The percentages of groups who would have gone to each town anyway were: King's Lynn 15%, Wisbech 27%, Swaffham 11% and Downham Market 5%. From this evidence we conclude that visiting the hospital at Wisbech is the most integrated with the everyday life of the community and visiting at Downham Market (Stow Hall Hospital) is the least integrated. This confirms our impressions based on the origins of in-patients and the locations of the hospitals with reference to the town centres. Overall, it appears that about 13% of visiting trips involve less effort, time and cost than might be surmised simply from the information given about the origin and duration of the journey. But the 13% of groups who would have visited the town anyway consist almost entirely of groups with their own means of transport. The 13% amounts to 20 trips, of which only one was by bus.

Town catchment areas

In planning the location of community hospitals in a rural district it is desirable to take account of the catchment areas of the towns that are possible sites. For many people living in the study district a visit to King's Lynn or Wisbech is likely to be a frequent event and for them a trip to a hospital or clinic in these towns is unlikely to be perceived as difficult. Other people will visit these towns much less often and are likely to perceive the journey as being much more difficult. Both the out-patients survey and the survey of visitors to preconvalescent and geriatric patients collected information on the frequency of trips made to towns in the King's Lynn District other than for hospital visiting purposes and this information gives an indication of the towns' general catchment areas.

Clearly, the ideal situation is one in which there is exact correspondence between the general catchment area of the town (for shopping and other purposes) and the catchment area of its hospital. Replies to the visitor survey show that there are large differences between places in the degree to which the ideal is approached: differences that have already been foreshadowed in the analysis of the home origins of the sample of in-patients.

When individual visitors were asked how often they came to the town other than to visit the hospital almost half of them (44%) indicated that they made weekly or more frequent visits to the town. For them a trip to the hospital involved a journey frequently made for other purposes (although it will be recalled that only a minority actually did other things while visiting hospital). The group included the 15% of visitors who lived in the same town as the hospital. At the other end of the scale, a similar proportion of visitors (43%) visited the town less than monthly, so for them the hospital visit was a marked variation in their normal movement pattern.

A breakdown according to the town where the hospital was situated is given in Table 4.29. The people who lived in the same town as the hospital they visited are not included. What is clear from the table

is that the visitors to hospital in Wisbech and Swaffham are much more
used to visiting those towns for other purposes than the visitors to
King's Lynn and, especially, Downham Market.   The percentages of
hospital visitors who made weekly or more than weekly trips for other
purposes to the same town are: Swaffham, 76%; Wisbech, 56%; King's
Lynn, 35% and Downham Market, a mere 14%.   This, of course, is as
much a reflection of the different sizes and functions of the hospitals
as of the general catchment areas of the towns.   Simply from the point
of view of visiting trips, the hospitals in Swaffham and Wisbech are a
much more integrated part of community life than are the hospitals of
King's Lynn and Downham Market.   Swaffham Cottage Hospital is already
close to the "community hospital" pattern.   The North Cambridgeshire
Hospital in Wisbech (in which most of the Wisbech sample was obtained)
is a general hospital that, because of its small size, is able to draw
most of its visitors from the people who regularly visit Wisbech.
The King's Lynn hospitals, on the other hand, take patients from an
area extending beyond the everyday influence of the town and this is
even more true of the preconvalescent outpost near Downham Market, which
is able to derive little benefit from the day to day activities and
movements within the district.

Table 4.29
Frequency of visitors' trips to town, by town

Frequency	King's Lynn %	Wisbech %	Downham %	Swaffham %
Daily	11	21	5	28
1-3 times weekly	24	35	9	48
1-3 times monthly	18	10	16	8
less often	47	34	70	16
BASE	45	68	120	25

The nature of the general catchment areas for the towns of King's
Lynn and Wisbech is shown more clearly by the larger sample of the out-
patients survey.   Table 4.30 illustrates that the frequency of trips
out-patient respondents made to these towns for purposes other than
visiting the hospital is closely related to how far away the respondents
lived from the town in question.   Within about eight miles, trips were
fairly frequent.   Most people living within this distance made a trip
of a least weekly frequency whereas very few people went less often
than monthly.   Beyond about eight miles, trip frequencies were much
lower.   It therefore seems that the catchment areas of King's Lynn and
Wisbech for regular trips are rather small, certainly much smaller
than the catchment areas of the out-patient clinics in the towns.

Table 4.30 confirms two general principles well known to geographers
and planners.   The first is that the extent of the catchment area or
sphere of influence of a town is related to the size of the town.
Since King's Lynn followed by Wisbech are the largest towns in the study
district, the areas of influence of the other towns will almost

certainly be more limited. The second principle is that a town's catchment area cannot be delineated by a line on a map, for the influence of a town does not stop at any particular distance but continues to diminish in a regular manner as distance from the town is increased. Thus, the towns in the King's Lynn District are surrounded not by their own distinct catchment areas but by probability fields that overlap at the edges. A further complication is revealed by breaking down the data in Table 4.30 to examine the habits of characteristic groups within the sample. When this was done, it was found that there were statistically significant tendencies for visits to town to be more frequent for people from car owning households, for those with driving licences and for younger adults. That is, exactly as was found earlier for multi-purpose trips, it was the more mobile groups in the sample that visited the towns more often. This suggests that the extent of the probability fields discussed above will differ for different groups. For more mobile groups the probability fields are likely to be more extensive, whereas, for the less mobile groups they are likely to be smaller. It is very difficult, then, to compare the catchment area of a hospital with the "catchment area" of a town. The message of Table 4.30 remains, however, that most frequent, non-hospital, trips to King's Lynn and Wisbech take place within a radius of eight or ten miles. People drawn into the hospitals from greater distances will generally be making an unaccustomed journey.

Table 4.30
Frequency of visits to town, by distance (out-patients sample)

| | King's Lynn | | Wisbech | |
	% weekly or more	% less than monthly	% weekly or more	% less than monthly
0-2 miles	91	4	86	7
2-4 miles	88	6	89	9
4-6 miles	66	16	80	14
6-8 miles	44	19	52	8
8-10 miles	29	46	21	47
10-12 miles	16	53	14	57
12-14 miles	16	39	-	-
Over 14 miles	7	74	-	-

SUMMARY

Three questionnaire surveys were carried out to investigate the costs and other inconveniences that patients and visitors incur in their trips to hospital. The first survey was of a sample of out-patients attending clinics. The second was of preconvalescent and geriatric in-patients considered suitable for care in a small local hospital and the people who visited them in hospital. The third survey was of elderly mentally infirm patients and their visitors.

While most patients and visitors included in the samples had travelled distances of only a few miles to hospital, a minority had journeys exceeding 20 miles. At very small distances from the hospital many out-patients and visitors went on foot, but for distances greater than two miles by far the most popular mode of transport was the private car. Most car users travelled to hospital in their own car but substantial proportions relied upon lifts given in someone else's car. Only 10% of out-patients and a tiny minority of in-patients (1%) and their visitors (3%) travelled by public transport. Those who did were often travelling within the towns. Public transport apparently does not provide a useful link to hospitals for rural dwellers who do not own a car.

The costs for a journey to hospital, both for the few who used public transport and the many who went by car, were generally not high. Most return trips cost less than £1, but some people did pay more. For them, and for the visitors who had modest but frequently occurring travel costs, travel to hospital is likely to have involved significant expenditure. The relationship between the cost of travel and the distance was examined from the replies of public transport users and an estimate of car running costs per mile was obtained. The association between journey time and distance was also examined. Using these relationships, a method was suggested for predicting average journey cost and time from a known distance.

For most out-patients and visitors the trip to hospital was a single purpose journey, but almost half the out-patients and about 10% of visitors were able to combine it with another activity such as going to work or shopping. Multi-purpose trips reduce the costs and inconvenience of the hospital journey for those who are able to make them, but those who are able to make them tend to be the younger, more mobile people living not far from the hospitals, for whom the trip is easy anyway. Many out-patients were found to need to make special arrangements at home or work when they attended the out-patient clinic, but it seems that the numbers needing to make such arrangements is likely to be only marginally affected by the location of clinics. Out-patients would still need to take time off work and would still need to make arrangements for children, for example, wherever the clinic is located. However, the length of time the patient is away from home or work would inevitably be related to the location of clinics, and some evidence was found that the need to be accompanied by another person was greater for longer journeys.

Examination of the addresses of the patients in the sample showed that the hospitals involved had very different catchment areas. Some drew their patients from a radius of only a few miles, others served the whole health district and the two psychiatric hospitals contained patients from more than one health district. The majority of visitors lived in the same parish as the patient they had come to visit, so the areas from which visitors were drawn corresponded quite closely to the patient catchment areas: a finding which enables visitors' trips to be estimated from the home locations of in-patients. The contrasting catchment areas for in-patients of different hospitals were reflected in the frequency with which visitors were in the habit of going to the town for purposes other than visiting the hospital. The hospitals with restricted in-patient catchment areas drew in many more visitors who were used to visiting the town regularly than did the hospitals with district-wide catchments.   In this sense the "local" hospitals were observed to have visiting patterns which conformed much more with the day to day life of the community than the hospitals which served a wider area.

The costs and inconveniences to patients and visitors reported here do not tell the whole story because they apply only to the people who actually made the trip to hospital.   Any potential patients who were not referred to hospital or any potential visitors who did not visit because of the inhibiting effect of distance were not represented in the results.   If any such people exist, then the rural community is incurring social costs subtler and perhaps more serious than those described so far.   We turn to this subject in the next chapter.

5 Distance, satisfaction and trip suppression

The most important advantage of the community hospital system compared
with a completely centralised district general hospital strategy is
that it offers a service that is more accessible to the community.
In the previous chapter the costs incurred by patients and visitors in
getting to hospital under the present system were identified and
related to accessibility, so that the effect of different distributions
of hospital beds might be estimated. Applied at its simplest, this
estimating procedure involves the assumption that the geographical
origins of patients and visitors will be the same whatever the
arrangement of hospitals : an improvement in accessibility means a
decrease in costs and a decrease in accessibility is matched by a
corresponding increase in costs, for the same people. But in reality
perhaps matters are not so simple. It may be, for example, that
people living close to hospitals and people who are relatively mobile
may be more likely to be referred to an out-patient clinic or be
admitted to hospital as an in-patient than immobile people living some
distance away. It certainly seems likely that the accessibility of
hospitals will affect whether or not visiting trips are made, so the
possibility must be allowed that different geographical arrangements
of hospital beds in a district could produce different patterns of
geographical origins of patients and visitors.

The purpose of this chapter is to examine the effects of distance
from hospital on out-patient attendances, in-patient admissions and
visiting rates. Evidence is drawn from surveys conducted in hospital
(surveys of out-patients, in-patients and visitors, together with
data on hospital discharges supplied by the health authority) and also
from information collected out of hospital, in the community.
Here we are as much concerned with the trips to hospital that are not
made as with those that are, and studies of the people who actually
arrive in hospital are in danger of missing the ones who stay at home.
We begin, then, with an account of a door-to-door survey of people
living in rural Norfolk, to explore whether remoteness has an effect
on hospital trips and to what extent anxieties about the hospital
service could be reduced by a careful hospital location policy.

ACCESSIBILITY AND SATISFACTION

The best access to hospitals in the King's Lynn Health District is
undoubtedly enjoyed by the residents of King's Lynn itself and Wisbech.
Generally speaking, the people who live away from these towns are at
a disadvantage, but it is not known to what extent this relative
disadvantage is accepted as being an inevitable part of living in the
country or whether it is a source of real discontent. If accessibility is a real issue, it ought to be possible to distinguish
differences in attitude between rural people who live relatively close

to the main towns and rural people living in the remoter parts.
Do the people who appear to be most at a disadvantage actually feel
most discontented? Furthermore, are the effects of inaccessibility
felt by some identifiable groups of people more than others?
To provide tentative answers to these questions a survey of attitudes
was carried out in a number of villages in north-west Norfolk.

The community survey

Interviews were conducted in twelve villages, divided into two groups.
One group was chosen to be representative of villages accessible to
King's Lynn with its concentration of medical and other services.
All of these villages were close to King's Lynn and had good bus
services to it. The other group was more distant from King's Lynn,
had generally poorer public transport connections and hence could be
regarded as being inaccessible (see Figure 5.1 and Table 5.1). Care
was taken to include both large and small villages in each group.

Table 5.1
Villages in the community survey

Village	Straight-line distance to King's Lynn (mls)	Number of buses to King's Lynn per week	Number of completed interviews
Accessible:			
Middleton	4	89	50
Wormgay	6	49	45
Tottenhill	6	49	20
Gayton	7	34	104
Hillington	7	20	20
Castle Rising	4	176	29
Inaccessible:			
Syderstone	15	3	40
Docking	14	18	53
Stanhoe	15	17	25
North Creake	18	2	56
Burnham Market	19	29	46
Burnham Thorpe	19	1	23

The survey was carried out during the evening of Wednesday 4 May
1977 by students from the University of East Anglia trained in social
survey techniques. Shortage of both time and money precluded the use
of a random sampling technique. Instead, each student was assigned a
part of a village and was instructed to complete a quota of interviews
with adults in a cross-section of the houses in his area. Only one
person per household was interviewed and 511 interviews were completed,
268 in "accessible" villages and 243 in "inaccessible" villages.
Table 5.1 shows the number in each village. The interview form is
given in Appendix G. Altogether, 97 interviews were refused.

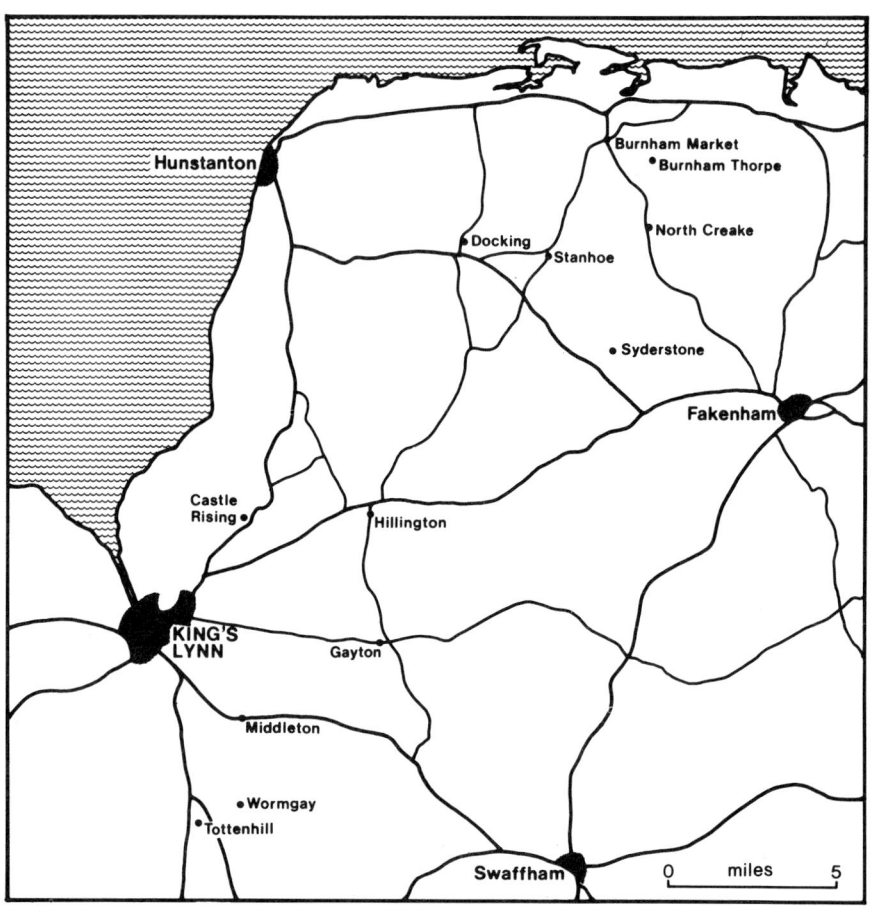

Figure 5.1   Location of villages for community survey

The representativeness of the sample was assessed by comparing the age, sex and social class composition of the sample with that of the population of the relevant parishes as reported in the 1971 census. Using the chi-square test at the 0.05 significance level, no differences were found between sample and population for both sex and social class composition. The measure of social class composition used was a crude division into "white collar workers" (socio-economic groups 1-7, 13 and 14) and "blue collar workers" (socio-economic groups 8-11 and 15). In terms of age structure, however, the sample was different from the 1971 population. The sample contained less people in the 16-44 age group (41% as opposed to 45%) and more people in the 65 and over age group (26% compared with 20%) than was expected from the 1971 census. These differences might be explained by changes in the age structure between 1971 and 1977. Comparison of the census figures of 1961 and 1971 for the west Norfolk rural area shows that during the period there was a marked increase in the proportion of elderly to younger persons which, if continued into the seventies, would account for the discrepancy. The level of household car ownership in the population has also changed since the 1971 census, but the sample figure of 78% is close to the estimate made for the district in Chapter 2. It seems, then, that the sample is representative in terms of sex, social class composition and car ownership levels and perhaps in terms of age structure as well.

Satisfaction with hospital services

The responses to a general question about the hospitals serving that part of Norfolk showed that most people were well pleased with the hospital service available. While 35% of respondents said they were "very satisfied" and 41% said they were "satisfied" with the hospitals serving the district, 8% were "neither satisfied nor dissatisfied", 5% were "dissatisfied" and only 3% were "very dissatisfied" (9% did not know). There were no marked differences in general satisfaction with hospitals between different groups in the population although there were slight tendencies (not statistically significant) for higher proportions to be satisfied amongst older people, women, blue-collar workers and non car-owners, and in the less accessible villages.

In addition to asking about satisfaction with the district's hospitals in general the survey also asked about satisfaction with a number of specific issues relating to hospitals. The issues were as follows:

(a) The length of time people who need an operation have to wait before being admitted to hospital

(b) The rules and regulations for patients in hospital

(c) The friendliness of hospitals

(d) The travelling for people who want to visit patients in hospital

(e) The amount of information given to patients about what is wrong with them

(f) The visiting hours

(g) The travelling time in getting patients to hospital in an emergency

(h)   Patients being cared for by doctors and nurses they have not met before

(i)   The travelling for people who have to get to hospital clinics

Table 5.2 shows the results of this section of the survey.   It demonstrates that there was a high level of satisfaction with many aspects of the hospital service but that a few did give rise to dissatisfaction.   People were generally satisfied with the rules and regulations for patients in hospital, with the friendliness of hospitals, with visiting hours, with their familiarity with hospital staff and with emergency travel to hospital.   For each of these issues less than 20 per cent of the respondents expressed dissatisfaction.   However, on two issues, "travel for visitors" and "waiting lists", there was a considerable degree of dissatisfaction, with the number dissatisfied exceeding the number satisfied.   Additionally, there was a somewhat lower degree of dissatisfaction expressed in respect of "information to patients" (about a quarter dissatisfied) and "travel to clinics" (about one third dissatisfied) although in each of these cases the numbers who were satisfied exceeded the numbers dissatisfied.

Table 5.2
Satisfaction with aspects of hospitals

Percentage who were:

	Very satisfied	Satisfied	Neither satisfied nor dissatisfied	Dissatisfied	Very dissatisfied	Don't know
Waiting lists	7	18	8	33	12	24
Rules and regulations	13	51	9	3	1	23
Friendliness	37	47	4	4	0	7
Travel for visitors	3	22	8	29	23	14
Information to patients	9	32	9	17	9	25
Visiting hours	21	59	4	4	0	12
Emergency travel	16	35	4	12	7	26
Familiar staff	12	47	14	6	1	20
Travel to clinics	6	35	7	22	13	17

The degree of dissatisfaction with an issue can be summarised by calculating the ratio of the number dissatisfied and very dissatisfied to the number satisfied and very satisfied.   A high ratio indicates a high level of dissatisfaction.   Interestingly, the source of dissatisfaction with the highest ratio was travelling to visit patients in hospitals.   It seems, then, that rural people do regard their lack of access to hospitals as a more serious disadvantage than other possible shortcomings in the service.   But was there greater dissatisfaction in the less accessible villages?   Table 5.3 confirms that this was

the case, with the inaccessible villages showing a ratio of dissatisfied to satisfied people almost twice that of the accessible
villages.

Table 5.3

Dissatisfaction with aspects of the hospital service in accessible
and inaccessible villages.

Issue	Ratio of dissatisfied to satisfied	
	Accessible Villages	Inaccessible villages
Travel for visitors*	1.53	2.92
Waiting lists*	2.45	1.36
Travel to clinics	0.98	0.74
Information to patients*	0.83	0.44

* = Difference between accessible and inaccessible villages in the
number of people either satisfied or dissatisfied is statistically
significant at the 0.05 level.

Table 5.3 also shows that for the other perceived shortcomings of
the hospital service the reverse was the case.   People in accessible
villages were less satisfied than their more remote counterparts with
the length of waiting lists, the travelling to get to clinics and the
amount of information given to patients about what is wrong with them.
The reason for this reversal is not clear.   One possibility is that
people in the remoter villages have lower expectations about quality.
Whatever the reason, the results are in line with a study of urban
and rural differences in the United States which found that whereas
rural people were more dissatisfied than urban people on the accessibility of health care, in general the rural people were more satisfied
with regard to the quality of care they received than the urban people
(Aday and Andersen, 1975).   Apparently, people with poor access to
health care emphasise that single complaint, while people with
relatively good access may have higher expectations concerning other
aspects of the service.   The reasons that travelling to clinics and
the travelling time in getting people to hospital in an emergency were
not emphasised as difficulties by the "remote" people may be that these
represented hypothetical rather than real difficulties, as not many
respondents would have recent experience of them.   This, however, is
speculation.

Dissatisfaction and personal characteristics

Whilst overall attitudes to the difficulty of travel for visitors might
differ between accessible and inaccessible villages, the degree of
dissatisfaction might not be the same for all sections of the population.   In particular, one would expect that the groups who would be
likely to suffer the greatest problems in visiting patients in hospital
would show the highest levels of dissatisfaction.   Thus, greater
problems might be anticipated for less mobile groups such as the old,

non car owners and women.   Table 5.4 shows that in the inaccessible areas the level of dissatisfaction increased with age such that there was a ratio of dissatisfied to satisfied people of almost 8 to 1 amongst the over 65's as compared with about 2 to 1 in the under 44 age group.   The results also show that in both accessible and inaccessible areas dissatisfaction was greater for women than men, so that the most adverse situation was experienced by women in the inaccessible areas.   Broadly the same picture was true for non car owners.   Both car owners and non car owners in inaccessible villages were more dissatisfied than their counterparts in the accessible villages, with the non car owners in inaccessible villages being by far the most adversely affected group.

Table 5.4
Satisfaction with "travel for visitors" by personal characteristics

| | Ratio of dissatisfied to satisfied | |
	Accessible villages	Inaccessible villages
Age:		
16 - 44 years	1.39 (86)	1.95 (65)
45 - 64 years	1.75 (66)	2.48 (73)
65+*	1.43 (51)	7.83 (53)
Sex:		
Males	1.32 (79)	1.97 (92)
Females*	1.67 (123)	4.56 (100)
Car ownership:		
Car*	1.38 (157)	2.51 (144)
No car	2.31 (43)	5.71 (47)

Note: number in sample in brackets
     * = Difference between accessible and inaccessible villages
       in the number of people either satisfied or dissatisfied
       is statistically significant at the 0.05 level.

It is therefore possible to show that not only is dissatisfaction with travel for visitors related to the accessibility of the villages to hospitals but also to the level of mobility of different groups in the population.   Our findings suggest that the greatest problems are faced by the old, by women and by non car owners, particularly when they live in relatively inaccessible villages.

The other major issue which generated a high level of dissatisfaction - hospital waiting lists - showed a completely different pattern. Dissatisfaction was greater in the more accessible areas, it was greater for younger people and was greater for car owners than for non car owners.   The only similarity with the previous issue was that women were more dissatisfied than men, but much more markedly so in the accessible villages.   Women in accessible villages were more dissatisfied with waiting lists than women in inaccessible villages : a difference that was statistically significant.   In general, the groups who are dissatisfied with the size of waiting lists are precisely those who are not concerned with travel.   Perhaps these

are articulate middle class people who are not necessarily in a worse
position than their working class counterparts but who are more prone
to express criticism on abstract issues.   This explanation, however,
is not supported by a disaggregation into "white" and "blue collar"
workers which showed that, in the inaccessible villages at least, the
"blue collar" people interviewed were more critical of waiting lists
than the "white collar" people.   It seems that the most that can be
suggested by way of explanation is that expectations of the hospital
service were greater among people who had the easiest access to them.
Dissatisfaction focussed on the waiting list issue wherever accessibility to hospital was not a serious problem.

Similar results to those for "waiting lists" emerged in respect of
the more minor issue of the amount of information given to patients.
Dissatisfaction was greater in the more accessible areas, greater for
younger people, for non car owners and for women.   For the other
relatively minor cause of dissatisfaction - travelling to hospital
clinics - the results were, as indicated previously, more indicative
of a general, "abstract" shortcoming than a disadvantage perceived to
be important by less mobile groups.   One might expect dissatisfaction
to be greater in the more inaccessible areas but this was not the case.
Dissatisfaction was higher in the accessible areas although not to a
statistically significant extent.   It was greater for the younger
age group and greater for women than men.   In the accessible areas,
dissatisfaction was greater for car owners than for non car owners.
However, in the inaccessible areas non car owners were more dissatisfied: a finding that slightly breaks the pattern.

The results show that the importance of different issues varies
from one type of person to another and from type of area to another.
It does seem clear, though, that the difficulty of visiting patients
in hospital is perceived as a more serious problem by people living
in the remoter villages than those living in more accessible villages.
In so far as a policy of dispersed small hospitals would increase the
number of people living in "accessible" villages relative to those in
remote places, it would appear to offer an improvement.   A real
cause of concern might be lessened by the establishment of community
hospitals but it could be replaced, of course, by other more abstract
dissatisfactions with the hospital service.

ACCESSIBILITY AND HOSPITAL USE

An important effect of community hospitals is that they may possibly
extend hospital care to some people in the remoter rural areas who
would otherwise be less likely to receive it from a hospital in the
district centre.   To estimate the significance of this effect it is
necessary to investigate whether accessibility at present produces a
discernable increase in hospital use.   In this section we search for
evidence to confirm or deny such an effect in the results of the
community survey, in Hospital Activity Analysis for the whole of the
Norfolk Health Area, and in the survey of out-patients.

Evidence from the community survey

While it has been established that the difficulty of visiting inpatients was a source of real dissatisfaction among residents of the more remote villages, whether the difficulty of travel inhibited their visiting has not yet been explored. In addition to being asked about their satisfaction with aspects of the hospital service, respondents in the community survey were asked: "Have you ever visited a patient in hospital?" and "How many visits have you made to patients in hospital in the last year?" The lack of any distinctive response from residents of the more inaccessible villages to the issues of travelling for emergency in-patients and out-patients attending clinics has already been noted, but the hypothesis that accessibility may affect hospital use was pursued further by asking respondents whether they had ever been a patient in hospital and whether they had ever been to hospital as an out-patient. These questions did not distinguish between experiences of hospitals while resident in the survey village and previous experiences of those who had moved into the study area, so the most that could be expected from the answers was a crude indication of the likely effects of rural accessibility.

At some stage in their lives most respondents in the community survey had been in-patients or out-patients and an overwhelming majority had visited someone in hospital (Table 5.5). Even considering only the past year a substantial proportion had visited someone in hospital. The survey revealed, then, a widespread use of hospitals.

Table 5.5
Percentage of respondents who had been in-patients, out-patients or visitors.

	Accessible villages %	Inaccessible villages %	All villages %
In-patients	68	61	65
Out-patients	70	63	67
Visitor : ever	90	87	89
Visitor : past year	46	39	42

When the respondents are divided into those living in accessible villages and those in inaccessible villages, Table 5.5 shows that people in the inaccessible villages were less likely to have been in-patients, out-patients or visitors to hospitals. Although none of these differences were strong enough to be statistically significant at the 0.05 level, the results are consistent in suggesting that accessibility may influence the use of hospitals. However, each of these measures of hospital use suffers from being based on the life-long experience of the respondent. Since population mobility is quite high one would expect this to blur any distinction between hospital usage in accessible and inaccessible areas. For example, some of the people interviewed in inaccessible areas might previously have lived in accessible areas and vice versa. One would expect, therefore, that the overall effect of population mobility would be to reduce the difference in usage rates between areas. Consequently if the survey had concentrated on long-term residents in each area the differences might have been greater than those observed. One item of information which suffers less from this problem is that of frequency of visiting during the past year. Table 5.5 shows that the frequency of visiting in the past year was higher in accessible than in inaccessible areas, thus confirming the differences observed for the lifelong data discussed above. It should be noted that for this shorter time span the differences between visiting rates for accessible and inaccessible areas were greater than for visiting rates on a lifelong basis.

Given that there were these differences between the two groups of villages, did they arise from differences in accessibility or were they simply the result of differences in the population structure of the two groups? For example, if one group had had more women than the other this would be expected to produce differences in the proportions who had been in-patients. Similarly, variations in the proportions of different age groups and variations in car ownership and socio-economic group structure might account for the observed differences between the two groups of villages. In an attempt to test for these effects the data were disaggregated by age, sex, car ownership and socio-economic group. Table 5.6 shows the results of these analyses. Since the past year data are probably more reliable than the whole-life data the former were used as the measure of visiting in these analyses.

Broadly speaking, the results confirm that even after disaggregation differences remained between the accessible and the inaccessible villages, although once again most differences were not statistically significant. The results also appear to indicate that the differences between the two groups of villages were not the same for all types of people. For example, the proportions of men who had been in-patients or who had been visitors in the past year did not differ between the two groups of villages. Similarly, out-patients and visiting rates varied little for the people aged 16-44 years. On the other hand, for certain groups, particularly for women and the elderly, the differences between accessible and inaccessible villages were quite great. In general it seems possible to conclude that the differences between accessible and inaccessible villages were greater for those groups in the population who tended to have low levels of mobility. On the other hand, younger people and men, whom one would expect to be more mobile, did not show such marked differences between the two types of area. Accessibility appears to be an important factor in determining the extent to which people use hospitals as in-patients, out-patients or visitors, but it seems that not all types of people are equally disadvantaged by living in areas remote from hospitals. It follows from this that a policy of dispersing hospitals would benefit certain groups to a greater extent than others.

Table 5.6
Experience of hospitals disaggregated by age, sex, socio-economic
group, car ownership and accessibility.

Sub-sample		In-patients %	Out-patients %	Visitors %	Number in sample
16 - 44 years	A	66	69	48	125
	INA	59	67	49	81
45 - 64 years	A	71	74	41	82
	INA	63	62	38	88
65+ years	A	66	69	47*	61
	INA	58	57	29*	69
Males	A	56	75*	38	109
	INA	56	59*	37	114
Females	A	76	67	50	157
	INA	66	65	40	125
Manual workers	A	69	72	49	116
	INA	61	67	40	105
Non-manual workers	A	68	68	54	69
	INA	62	66	35	48
Car owning	A	69*	71	47	213
	INA	59*	61	41	182
Non car owning	A	62	65	37	52
	INA	67	64	27	57

Note: A = Accessible villages   INA = Inaccessible villages
       * = Difference between accessible and inaccessible villages
           in the number of people with or without hospital
           experience is statistically significant at the 0.05 level

Hospital Activity Analysis data

The possibility that people living in relatively remote Norfolk
villages were less likely to be admitted as in-patients than similar
people living in more accessible villages was considered serious
enough to merit further investigation, so data relating hospital use
to area of residence were obtained from the East Anglian Regional
Health Authority.   The data used were Hospital Activity Analysis
tabulations of the number of discharges during 1976 from all East
Anglian hospitals to the 31 former local authority areas within the
Norfolk Health Area.   The local 'authority areas comprised 15 urban
areas (county boroughs, municipal boroughs and urban districts) and
16 rural districts.   Psychiatric, maternity and day patients were not
included in the data.   To provide a standard of comparison, the
expected number of discharges for each local authority area was
calculated by applying national age and sex specific rates of discharge from Table 12 of the 1973 Hospital In-patient Enquiry (DHSS

and OPCS, 1975) to the age/sex composition of the local population derived from the 1971 population census. A ratio of the actual to the
expected number of discharges for each area was then calculated.

This procedure revealed substantial variations between areas in the
ratio of actual to expected numbers of discharges in the year, the
highest ratio being 153% greater than the lowest. Urban areas, with
an average ratio of 1.15, tended to have higher ratios than rural areas,
whose average was 0.81. A "t" test confirmed that the difference
between the means of the urban and rural samples was statistically
significant at the 0.05 level.

What are the reasons for this difference? Since most hospital beds
in the area are in towns the difference might be related to the greater
accessibility of hospitals to urban residents. If this were the case
one would expect the ratio of actual to expected discharges to be
higher in the rural areas which are close to the main towns than in the
rural areas which are more remote. To test this, the rural areas
were divided into two groups. The "accessible" group comprised
rural districts which had a boundary with one of the three main towns
in the study area, King's Lynn, Norwich and Great Yarmouth. The "less
accessible" group comprised those rural districts without such a
boundary. The average ratios were found to be 0.75 for the accessible areas and 0.84 for the less accessible areas: a tendency opposite
to the one which would be expected if accessibility to the main towns
was an important factor. The less accessible rural areas tended to
have higher ratios of actual to expected discharges (although this
difference was not statistically significant at the 0.05 level).

It can therefore be concluded that there is no evidence in the
Hospital Activity Analysis data to suggest that accessibility to
hospitals influences variations in hospital use from one rural district
to another. Furthermore, correlation analysis showed that neither
variations in social structure (as measured by the percentage of manual
workers in the population, from the 1971 census) nor variations in
health, measured by standardised mortality rates (Registrar General,
1975), were significantly associated with the ratios of actual to
expected discharges (the correlation coefficients were 0.23 and -0.01
respectively).

Why, then, did urban areas have significantly more in-patients than
rural areas whilst the remoter rural districts did not fare worse than
accessible rural districts? Work reported by Ashley (1972) makes it
seem likely that the answer lies in coding errors relating to area of
residence in the original Hospital Activity Analysis returns. All
correct postal addresses include the name of a post town, which is a
postal clearing point for a particular district. Thus, even people
living in remote rural districts include the name of a post town
perhaps several miles distant in their address. The danger is that
the patient's place of residence may be incorrectly recorded as the
post town rather than the rural district. Ashley's analysis of
hospital admission rates per thousand population in East Anglia
confirmed that urban districts in general had much higher admission
rates than rural districts, but when urban districts were divided into
those containing post towns and those not, a different picture emerged.

While the post town urban districts had the highest rates, the average rate for urban districts not containing a post town was lower than that for the rural districts. In the present study, all 15 urban areas were post towns. Of the 16 rural districts, three contained post towns. These three districts had an average actual to expected in-patient ratio of 0.87. The average ratio for the remaining rural districts was 0.79.

The conclusion from the somewhat suspect Hospital Activity Analysis data is that in 1976 at least the outlying rural population did not have lower in-patient admission rates than the rural population living closer to urban centres. (The analysis was based on hospital discharges but discharges can be regarded as being almost synonymous with admissions.) The implication is that community hospitals in the smaller urban centres would not increase the chances of a rural person being admitted as an in-patient. This conclusion contradicts that based upon the community survey, which itself was supported by the finding that rural general practitioners in the study district did report significantly lower satisfaction with the ease of admitting certain types of patient to hospital than the town-based general practitioners (Chapter 3). With the conflicting evidence available it seems that the effect of accessibility on in-patient admission warrants further attention in future.

The effect of accessibility on out-patients

The community survey indicated that inaccessibility may produce a negative effect on out-patient admission rates, but its similar indication of an effect on in-patients was not corroborated by the health service data. Out-patients, of course, are not included in the Hospital Activity Analysis, so it is not possible to use health service computer records to investigate the effect of distance from hospital on out-patient attendance. Here, we use our own out-patient survey to make further comments on the issue.

The method used was to compare actual and expected numbers of out-patients at different distances from King's Lynn. Actual numbers for each parish were derived from the survey data on trip origins. Expected numbers were calculated for each parish or town based on its population at the 1971 census, taking into account its age and sex distribution. Age/sex specific out-patient attendance rates for 1972 were derived from Table C11 of the Report of the Resource Allocation Working Party (DHSS, 1976). Both actual and expected numbers of out-patients were aggregated into three distance bands: those within King's Lynn, those outside King's Lynn but within ten miles and those more than ten miles away from King's Lynn. In the western part of the district the numbers attending out-patient clinics in King's Lynn were affected by the existence of clinics in Wisbech. To eliminate this effect from the analysis all parishes to the west of the River Ouse were excluded. However, this did not totally eliminate the influence of out-patient clinics outside of King's Lynn. Some out-patients from the district were likely to attend clinics in other towns, for example in Norwich. This was particularly so for those in the outer parts of the district for whom a trip to King's Lynn was only a little shorter than a trip to Norwich. Since the survey collected data in King's

Lynn, low numbers from these outlying parts might indicate not that these areas generated few out-patients but that many of them attended clinics outside King's Lynn.   Unfortunately we have no data which would allow us to measure the extent of such effects.   They should, however, be borne in mind when interpreting the results of the analysis.

Table 5.7 shows the actual distribution of out-patients recorded in the survey and the distribution one would expect on the basis of the age/sex weighted population living within various distances of King's Lynn.

Table 5.7
Actual and expected distribution of out-patients by distance from King's Lynn.

Distance from King's Lynn in miles	Actual %	Expected %	Ratio of actual to expected
Within King's Lynn	45	27	1.67
10 miles or less	26	24	1.08
More than 10 miles	29	49	0.59

In King's Lynn itself there were more out-patients than might be expected.   For places up to 10 miles from King's Lynn there were slightly more than expected.   Beyond 10 miles there were far fewer. Even bearing in mind the qualification discussed above these results suggest that proximity has a marked effect on the use which is made of out-patient clinics.   People living near to clinics are much more likely to use them than are people living at greater distances. Decisions on the location of clinics are, on the basis of this evidence, likely to affect who will benefit from them.

DISTANCE AND VISITING FREQUENCIES

One of the aims of the community hospital policy is to facilitate visiting for the relatives and friends of certain types of patient by making it possible for patients to be admitted to local rather than distant hospitals.   In order to estimate the likely effects of different community hospital strategies it is necessary not only to confirm that increasing the distances over which admissions are made causes visiting rates to be reduced, but also to quantify the relationship so that visiting rates may be predicted from in-patient home distances.   This is complicated by the fact that visiting rates are also associated with length of stay.   The relationship between visiting rates and distance in a set of data can only be isolated after first untangling the connection between visiting rates and length of stay.

Visiting rates and length of stay

Patients interviewed in the surveys of in-patients who had been in
hospital for longer than one week were asked how many different
visitors they received during the week up to the interview.   In the
survey of elderly mentally infirm patients, the ward sister or charge
nurse was asked to estimate the number of different visitors the
patient received in a typical month.   A further question identified
how many of the visitors were ministers of the church, social workers,
etc., and these visitors were excluded from the analysis.   Table 5.8
gives the percentage of preconvalescent and geriatric patients report-
ing varying numbers of different visitors.   The most frequently
reported number of different visitors was two.   Only 3% of preconvalescent patients, but 12% of geriatric patients, who had been in
hospital for more than one week had not been visited by anyone.
A surprising 3% of preconvalescent patients said they had been visited
by more than 20 different people in the past week.

Table 5.8
Number of different visitors received in one week

Number of visitors	Preconvalescent patients %	Geriatric patients %
0	3	12
1-5	45	63
6-10	35	20
11-15	11	5
16-20	3	0
Over 20	3	0
BASE	63	41

As much lower levels of visiting were experienced by the elderly
mentally infirm patients, the period of time for which an estimate was
made was lengthened to one month.   Altogether 35% of these patients
received no visitors during such a period (although there was evidence
of intermittent visiting - usually annually or twice a year - for about
one third of these).   One or two different visitors were received by
44% of elderly mentally infirm patients, 16% received three to five
visitors and 5% received between six and ten visitors.   These percentages are based on a total of 225 patients for whom estimates were
possible.

When they had recalled how many different people had come to visit
them in the past week or month, patients (or staff) were asked how
many times each of these visitors had come in that period.   The
number of visitor trips was calculated from replies to both questions:
that is, it refers to the number of different visitors multiplied by
the number of visits each.   Thus, a total of six visitor trips might
be made up of six different people each visiting once, three people
each visiting twice, or any other combination giving a product of six.

Table 5.9 gives the percentage of preconvalescent and geriatric patients receiving different numbers of visitor trips per week. The most frequently reported category was 11-15 visitor trips for preconvalescent patients and 1-5 visitor trips for geriatric patients.

Table 5.9
Total number of visitor trips received in one week

Number of visitor trips	Preconvalescent patients %	Geriatric patients %
0	3	12
1-5	11	54
6-10	20	17
11-15	25	7
16-20	15	3
Over 20	26	7

Similar information for elderly mentally infirm patients is presented in Table 5.10. For them the most frequently reported category was less than one visitor trip per month.

Table 5.10
Total number of visitor trips received by elderly mentally infirm patients in one month

Number of visitor trips	% of patients
0	38
1-2	23
3-5	16
6-10	13
Over 10	10

So far, visiting rates have been described only for patients who had been in hospital for more than one week. As Table 5.11 shows, 70% of the preconvalescent patients had been in hospital for less than seven complete days when the interview was conducted. Only 7% of geriatric patients were in this category, however. The elderly mentally infirm patients were characterised by much longer lengths of stay. While only 10% had been admitted within the previous month, 14% had been in hospital for 1-6 months, a further 14% for 6 months to one year and 62% for over one year.

Table 5.11
Length of stay in hospital before interview

Length of stay	Preconvalescent patients %	Geriatric patients %
0 days	8	0
1-3 days	40	5
4-6 days	22	2
1-4 weeks	24	16
1-3 months	5	19
Over 3 months	1	58
BASE	211	43

For preconvalescent and geriatric patients, visiting rates were
certainly affected by length of stay.   The pattern is illustrated in
Table 5.12 which gives the average number of visitor trips per day
according to length of stay.   The measure of average used is the
median rather than the mean because the distributions are highly
skewed : that is, the arithmetical mean would be inflated by a few
very high values.   For each length of stay category, the number of
visitor trips per day was calculated for every patient by dividing his
total number of visitor trips by the number of complete days he had
been in hospital (or by seven, if length of stay exceeded one week).
The median number of visitor trips per day was then identified for
each length of stay category and these are the numbers that appear in
the table.   For both types of patient the average daily number of
trips decreased markedly over long stays.   The sub-sample sizes are
too low to place reliance on the averages for geriatric patients with
less than one weeks' stay, but the much larger sample size makes it
possible to analyse the averages for short-term preconvalescent
patients in more detail than is shown in Table 5.12.   The median
number of visitor trips per day for preconvalescent patients increased
during the first part of the week from a total of two trips for
patients with one day's stay to four for those who had been in hospital
for four days.   Thereafter, the number declined.

Table 5.12
Median number of visitor trips per day by length of stay

Length of stay:	1-3 days	4-6 days	1-4 weeks	Over 4 weeks
Median trips per day:				
Preconvalescent patients	2	3	2	1
Geriatric patients	3*	2*	2*	0

* Based on less than 10 patients

As well as influencing the number of visitor trips per day to be expected by a patient, length of stay also affected the number of different visitors.   For the first few days of a stay in hospital, a patient may have expected to receive an increasing cumulative number as time passed, which reached a peak in the latter part of the week. For patients who had been in hospital for more than a month, the median number of different visitors dropped.   The figures for pre-convalescent and geriatric patients are compared in Table 5.13, but the geriatric figures should be treated with great caution as they are based on very small sub-samples.

Table 5.13
Median number of different visitors by length of stay

Length of stay:	1-3 days	4-6 days	1-4 weeks	Over 4 weeks
Median different visitors:				
Preconvalescent patients	3	5	6 (per week)	4(per week)
Geriatric patients	4*	10*	6* (per week)	3(per week)

* Based on less than 10 patients

It must be emphasised that these findings are the result of inter-viewing patients who were at different stages in their hospital stay. Some of the patients who were interviewed only a short time after admission may later have become longer-stay patients, but we have no direct evidence to suggest that their visitors would visit less frequently as time went on.   It may be the case that long stay patients tend to receive less visitors than short stay patients even in the first days after admission.   The results of the survey do not illuminate the development of visiting to a single patient as his stay becomes longer, but they do show that preconvalescent and geriatric patients who have been in hospital for different lengths of time experience different visiting patters.

Visiting rates for elderly mentally infirm patients showed a much less consistent pattern.   The length of stay categories used were: less than one month, one to six months, six months to one year and over one year.   Within these categories, the median numbers of visitor trips per month were: 2.5, 2, 4 and 1.   These figures show a decrease over the long term, but the peak in the six months to one year period is unaccountable except by reference to possible peculiar-ities in the subsample.   The average number of different visitors per month for elderly mentally infirm patients remained constant over time at a figure of 1, except again for the six months to one year period, for which a median of 1.5 was recorded.   It appears that visiting levels for elderly mentally infirm patients are so low that trends with time are less perceptible.

Visiting rates and distance

As well as being related to length of stay, visiting rates were found
to vary with distance. With increasing distance from the patient's
home to the hospital, patients generally received less visitor trips
and less different visitors (Tables 5.14 and 5.15). This appears to
be because a substantial proportion of visitors to patients lived
near the patient's home and consequently faced a long journey if the
patient was admitted to a distant hospital. Once again, the trends
were much weaker for elderly mentally infirm patients than for preconvalescent and geriatric patients. Indeed, no trend at all was
observable in the number of different visitors received by elderly
mentally infirm patients from varying distances.

Table 5.14
Median number of visitor trips by patient's home distance

Home distance:	0-2 miles	2-10 miles	10-20 miles	Over 20 miles
Median trips per day:				
Preconvalescent patients	3	3	2	2
Geriatric patients	1	1	0.5	0*
Elderly mentally infirm +	2	2	2	1

* Based on less than 10 patients
+ Median visitor trips per <u>month</u>

Table 5.15
Median number of different visitors by patient's home distance

Home distance:	0-2 miles	2-10 miles	10-20 miles	Over 20 miles
Median different visitors				
Preconvalescent patients	5.5	5	4	3
Geriatric patients	3	4.5	3.5	0.5*
Elderly mentally infirm +	1	1	1	1

* Based on less than 10 patients
+ Based on estimates for one month

Both these tables show the effect of distance but ignore the
parallel effect of length of stay on visiting. Equally, the pre-
ceeding Tables 5.12 and 5.13 ignore the effect of distance. The
combined effects of both variables are summarised by the median
values representing each length of stay and distance combination, as
in Table 5.16, where the median numbers of different visitors to preconvalescent patients are presented. Table 5.16 shows that time and
distance had a similar power in discouraging visitors. Within any
distance zone, the number of different visitors expected within one

week was reduced by up to half, on the average, by increasing the
length of stay from 1-4 weeks to over 4 weeks. Conversely, within
any length of stay period, the number of different visitors expected
was diminished by about the same margin as the patient's home distance
increased from 0-2 miles to over 20 miles. There is therefore a very
great difference observable when the two effects work together. For
example, a patient living less than two miles from the hospital who
had been in hospital for two weeks might have expected to receive an
average of ten different people as visitors, whereas a patient of six
weeks' duration, over twenty miles from home, might have received only
3 different visitors on average.

Table 5.16
Median number of different visitors to preconvalescent patients
by distance and length of stay

Length of stay:	1-3 days	4-6 days	1-4 weeks	Over 4 weeks
0-2 miles	5	6*	10 (per week)	6* (per week)
2-10 miles	3	8	7 "	8* "
10-20 miles	2	5	6 "	3* "
Over 20 miles	2.5	5*	4.5* "	3* "

* Based on less than 10 patients

One of the difficulties in disaggregating visiting data according to
two independent variables, as is done in Table 5.12, is that the data
are spread very thinly. Some distance and length of stay categories
contained so few patients that their average visiting rates cannot be
relied upon. This was especially the case for geriatric patients
(who were sparsely represented in the shorter length of stay categories) and for elderly mentally infirm patients (for the same reason),
so that tables relating median numbers of different visitors to
distance and length of stay are of doubtful validity and are not
included.

From the point of view of the patient, the number of different
people visiting appears likely to be less important than the total
visits he receives. Attention will therefore be concentrated on the
second measure. For preconvalescent patients, the evidence of
Table 5.17 is that the average number of visitor trips per day was
equally a function of length of stay and distance. Within all four
distance categories the number of visitor trips per day declined as
length of stay increased, and for any given length of stay period the
number of visitor trips per day decreased with increasing distance.
The average number of visitor trips per day for a 1-3 day patient
who lived in the same town as the hospital was 3.5, which contrasts
sharply with the average of one visitor per day for a patient admitted from over 20 miles away more than one month previously. The
table also shows how the deleterious effects of long stays may be
partially compensated for by a short patient home distance. While
two visitor trips per day was the norm for a patient admitted only
1-3 days previously and living 10-20 miles away, exactly the same
norm applied to the average patient hospitalised in his home town

131

for 1-4 weeks.

Table 5.17
Median number of visitor trips per day to preconvalescent patients
by distance and length of stay

Length of stay:	1-3 days	4-6 days	1-4 weeks	Over 4 weeks
0-2 miles	3.5	3.5	2	1.5*
2-10 miles	3	3	3	2*
10-20 miles	2	2	1.5	1.5*
Over 20 miles	1.5	3*	1.5*	1*

* Based on less than 10 patients

Because of the data difficulties outlined earlier, the corresponding table for geriatric patients (Table 5.18) is less informative.
In spite of gaps and inadequacies, however, it does appear to be
transmitting the same message: that over the range of data represented,
length of stay and the inpatient's home distance are both equally
strongly associated with the suppression of visitor trips. If this
is the case (and the evidence here is decidedly weaker than that for
preconvalescent patients) then hospital location policy would certainly
have an effect on the volume of visits made to geriatric patients.

Table 5.18
Median number of visitor trips per day to geriatric patients by
distance and length of stay

Length of stay:	1-3 days	4-6 days	1-4 weeks	Over 4 weeks
0-2 miles	4*	-	1*	0.5*
2-10 miles	-	2*	1.5*	0*
10-20 miles	2*	-	2*	0
Over 20 miles	-	-	-	0*

* Based on less than 10 patients

While hints of the same pattern may be discerned in the data for
elderly mentally infirm patients, the relationships between visiting,
length of stay and distance appear to be still weaker (if they are
present at all) for this in-patient group (Table 5.19). What appears
to be happening is that for patients who receive relatively large
numbers of visitors there is the opportunity, so to speak, for distance
and length of stay to produce marked effects. At the other end of
the scale, visiting for elderly mentally infirm patients appears to be
so close to the absolute minimum that the observable effects are
small. Visiting for geriatric patients appears to be in between these
extremes.

Table 5.19

Median number of visitor trips per month to elderly mentally infirm patients by·distance and length of stay

Length of stay	Under 1 month	1-6 months	6 months-1 year	Over 1 year
0-2 miles	2*	6*	4*	2
2-10 miles	2*	1	4*	2
10-20 miles	4*	0*	1.5*	2
Over 20 miles	1*	2	2	0

* Based on less than 10 patients

The indication that distance may affect visiting rates for relatively short stay geriatric patients does not appear to agree with that of a similar study conducted a few years ago. Investigating visiting rates to a sample of geriatric patients in hospitals in rural Shropshire, Cross and Turner (1974) concluded that whereas the duration of hospital stay had a pronounced effect upon visiting, for patients who had been in hospital for less than six months no effects of distance were discernable. Cross and Turner went on to recommend that relatively short stay geriatric patients could be accommodated within any distance up to 32 km from their homes without influencing visiting rates. A distance effect was, however, observable for geriatric patients whose stay exceeded six months.

Because of the different nature of our results and the importance of the issue in terms of community hospital policy we have subjected our data to statistical testing. Excluding those patients whose length of stay exceeded one year or who were admitted from outside the Health District, the information for the remaining geriatric patients was entered into a multiple regression analysis. This technique was used to find the best mathematical description of the relationship between the number of visitor trips per day, time in hospital and distance. The following non-linear equation was found to be the best fitting description:

$$V = 4.578 \frac{D^{0.0043}}{T^{0.4111}} \qquad (5.1)$$

where V was the number of visitor trips per day, D was the distance from the patient's home to the hospital in miles and T was the number of complete days the patient had been in hospital. (The coefficients were estimated by applying linear multiple regression to the logarithms of the variables).

The equation may be interpreted as saying that while the length of stay had a measurable negative effect on visiting for geriatric patients, on the average, distance had a negligible but slightly positive effect. The multiple correlation coefficient was not high (R=0.63), indicating that any attempt to predict the number of visitors per day for a particular patient would be likely to be highly inaccurate, but this comes as no surprise. What we are more interested in here is establishing whether or not an average relationship exists. That question is answered by significance tests on the multiple correlation coefficient (found to be significant at the 0.01 level), the partial regression coefficient of T (also significant at the 0.01 level) and the partial regression coefficient of D (not significant at the .05 level). That is to say, we can state with 99% confidence that the number of visitor trips to geriatric patients decreased with length of stay, but no dependable association with distance was shown by the data. We must, then, agree with the conclusion of Cross and Turner. Table 5.20 gives the number of visiting trips for various distances and lengths of stay which are predicted by the regression equation. Table 5.20 should, therefore, be compared with Table 5.18.

Table 5.20
Estimated number of visitor trips per day to geriatric patients by distance and length of stay

Length of stay:	2 days	1 week	2 weeks	6 weeks
1 mile	3.4	2.0	1.5	0.9
6 miles	3.5	2.1	1.6	0.9
15 miles	3.5	2.1	1.6	0.9
25 miles	3.5	2.1	1.6	0.9

A rather different conclusion was reached after applying the same type of analysis to the data for preconvalescent patients. The equation which was found to offer the best description of the relationship was:

$$V = \frac{4.115}{D^{0.1872} T^{0.1863}} \qquad (5.2)$$

where V was the number of visitor trips per day, D was the distance from the patient's home to the hospital in miles and T was the number of complete days the patient had been in hospital.

In this equation, both distance and time in hospital have a negative effect on visiting. The multiple correlation coefficient was very low (R=0.37), but a significance test on it was positive at the 0.001 level. In other words, we can be 99.9% confident that there is a true relationship and not just a random association between the three variables investigated of the number of visitor trips, length of stay and distance. The partial regression coefficients were both significant at better than the 0.001 level, showing that distance and time were each contributing separately to diminishing visiting rates.

The number of visitor trips per day which, on the average, preconvalescent patients with different lengths of stay and home to hospital distances might expect are given in Table 5.21. These numbers have been derived by applying the multiple regression equation. Distances of 1 mile, 6 miles, 15 miles and 25 miles together with lengths of stay of 2 days, 1 week, 2 weeks and 6 weeks, have been used to make the table comparable with Table 5.17, but any other combinations (within the range of the data) can readily be evaluated simply by substituting the appropriate numbers in the equation.   Table 5.21 shows quite clearly the average inhibitory effects of both time and distance working together.   This information will be directly useful in the evaluation stage of the community hospital planning study when a mechanism for estimating the numbers of visitors expected for large numbers of in-patients will be required.

Table 5.21
Estimated number of visitor trips per day to preconvalescent patients by distance and length of stay

Length of stay	2 days	1 week	2 weeks	6 weeks
1 mile	3.6	2.9	2.5	2.1
6 miles	2.6	2.0	1.8	1.5
15 miles	2.2	1.7	1.5	1.2
25 miles	2.0	1.6	1.4	1.1

SUMMARY

The subject of this chapter was the effect of distance from hospital on people's use of and satisfaction with hospital services.   The investigation used information from a door-to-door survey of people living in rural Norfolk, surveys of out-patients and people visiting hospital in-patients and Hospital Activity Analysis data on the origins of in-patients.

The results of the community survey showed that generally the people interviewed were satisfied with the hospitals of the area but there were certain more specific issues which caused considerable dissatis-faction.   The greatest problem was the difficulty of travel to visit patients in hospital.   This problem was perceived much more acutely in the remoter villages and by those groups in the population likely to have relatively low personal mobility.   The second most important issue giving rise for concern was that of the length of waiting lists. In contrast, this issue caused greater dissatisfaction amongst those people likely to have relatively high levels of personal mobility, particularly those in villages accessible to hospitals.   Other issues concerned with access - the travelling necessary to get to hospital clinics and the travel time in getting patients to hospital in emergency - were sources of dissatisfaction for some people, but not a majority and not especially for people who lived in the remoter villages.   It appears, then, that the difficulty of visiting patients is the most acutely felt access problem.   There is some evidence to suggest that as access is improved, the receding dominance of the transport problem is counterbalanced by an increase in other complaints stemming from higher expectations.

The community survey also furnished some indications (too weak to be statistically significant) that people in relatively remote villages were less likely to use hospitals than those living in relatively accessible villages. The proportions of people amongst those interviewed who had been in-patients, out-patients or who had visited other people in hospital were marginally less in the remote villages. Again, women and the elderly appeared to be slightly more at a disadvantage than men and younger people. These tentative conclusions were not, however, supported by scrutiny of Hospital Activity Analysis tabulations of discharges from East Anglian hospitals to Norfolk local authority areas in 1976. According to the health service records, the highest hospital discharge rates were to urban areas, followed by the relatively inaccessible rural areas. The relatively accessible rural areas had the lowest discharge rates. It was not possible to explain these differences using variations in social structure or health, but it did seem likely that they were the products of the incorrect coding of postal addresses in the Hospital Activity Analysis. A relationship between accessibility and in-patient admission rates remains a possibility, but it has not been demonstrated by the evidence available. Because out-patients are not represented in the Hospital Activity Analysis it was not possible to check our tentative findings concerning this group against health service data. A study of the home addresses of respondents in the out-patient survey, though, did reveal that lower rates of attendance were associated with greater distances from the clinic. It does seem likely, then, for out-patients if not for in-patients, that the geographic distribution of hospital services influences to a slight extent which particular patients are referred.

An often-mentioned advantage of small, local hospitals is that they facilitate visiting, but the extent to which the actual frequency of visiting is controlled by the ease of access was not known. The results presented here showed that in some cases both the number of different visitors received and the total numbers of visits were affected not only by the length of stay of the patient but also by the distance of the hospital from the patient's home. The relationship varied considerably in strength between different types of in-patient. The elderly mentally infirm patients in our sample experienced extremely low visiting rates (with an average of one visitor and two visitor trips per month) and contained such little variation that it was possible to distinguish neither a length of stay nor a distance effect. Visiting to geriatric patients was much more frequent. The averages were three different visitors and three visitor trips per week. While the average numbers of visits received by geriatric patients in different length of stay and distance categories suggested that both variables were effective in reducing visiting, further statistical analysis confirmed only the influence of length of stay as being significant. For preconvalescent patients, however, a highly significant association between visiting and both time and distance was shown. On the average, preconvalescent patients received fourteen visitor trips (comprising six different visitors) per week, but these averages changed in a predictable manner according to the length of stay and home distance characteristics of the patient. An algebraic expression was derived from the data to describe such changes. This, together with the other findings on the effects of distance, will be incorporated into a technique for evaluating some of the consequences of different hospital location policies.

6 The implications of different community hospital locations

It is the conventional wisdom that a dispersed network of small local hospitals would be expensive for the health service but advantageous for the community. However, the order of magnitude of the supposed costs and benefits has not been clearly established. If a health authority must decide between, say, two or three community hospitals for a district, by how much will costs to the health service increase and those to the community decrease as the number is raised from two to three? Similarly, if the choice is between a single hospital in place A or a hospital in place B, what are the implications of these altern- ative locations for both the providers and the users of the service? Such comparisons are the only basis for reasoned planning policy, yet in practice they are made in a rather one-sided manner. Health authorities are in a position to provide detailed estimates of the internal costs likely to be incurred under various policy options. These estimates are, of course, inevitably founded on a series of assumptions, some of which may turn out to be false, so their accuracy cannot be guaranteed, but they remain the best estimates possible with current knowledge. When it comes to the implications for the community, however, the estimates that can be provided are much more sketchy and may even be limited to a single map of travel times from hospital. There is no commonly accepted method for measuring the different facets of accessibility of the population to health care facilities. In this chapter we attempt to partially redress the situation by suggesting a method and demonstrating it in the study area.

Different community hospital strategies might be expected to have various costs and benefits to the community but, as was made clear in Chapter 1, this study concentrates on those associated with accessi- bility and travel. The method for estimating the accessibility implications of different hospital location strategies consists, first, of establishing the most probable geographical distribution of patients and their visitors and, second, measuring the distances of people to hospitals and drawing inferences about modes of transport, costs and times. For the first stage the source of information is the small area statistics from the 1971 census of population, modified by age-sex specific rates of bed usage or out-patient attendance. The second stage relies heavily upon extrapolations made from our own surveys in the King's Lynn Health District. It need hardly be said that the 1971 census is now out of date and the surveys were based on small samples in only one part of the country. Nevertheless, the information used is thought to be the best available. Population estimates are regularly brought up to date and projections into the future are made, but the basic information about the age and sex composition of small areas remains the latest census. For the relationships discovered in the surveys we do not claim universal validity: they are no more than estimates of general trends, but as such they are useful. The results produced are heavily dependent upon the assumptions made, but it is not possible to avoid making assumptions in any estimation procedure.

It is the general approach rather than its specific results that we wish to emphasise, and the general approach is flexible enough to incorporate different assumptions if there are doubts about the validity of the original ones or if new information becomes available.

This chapter first describes the construction of the estimating methods which are referred to as "models". Using the models, different hospital location strategies in the King's Lynn Health District were evaluated for out-patients and for three groups of in-patients (preconvalescent, geriatric and elderly mentally infirm) and their visitors. The results of the evaluations are presented in the second section. Finally, a simplified estimation procedure is described and its effectiveness is compared with that of the more complex method.

THE STRUCTURE OF THE MODELS

The estimation methods for out-patients, in-patients and visitors all used the parish, municipal borough or urban district as the basic areal unit. There are 158 parishes and urban areas in the King's Lynn Health District and, for the sake of convenience, all of them will be referred to as "parishes". Computer programs were written to process the parish data and to perform a series of calculations on them. The mechanics of these operations will be described for each model in turn.

Out-patients model

The stages of the out-patients model were as follows:

(1) Establish the various strategies of clinic locations to be eval-uated.

(2) Calculate the expected share of each parish in the district's out-patient attendances.

(3) Estimate the expected number of out-patient attendances per year from each parish.

(4) Assign all out-patients to their nearest clinic, under each strategy.

(5) Calculate the distances to be travelled.

(6) Repeat stages 3-5, assuming that distance affects the number of attendances.

(7) Estimate the modes of transport used.

(8) Estimate the trip costs and times.

Each of these stages requires explanation. As the first stage, a total of nine location strategies were chosen to illustrate the range of policy options from complete centralisation on the one hand to considerable dispersion on the other. Thus, the first strategy involved one clinic in King's Lynn, the ninth included clinics in King's Lynn, Wisbech, Swaffham, Downham Market and Hunstanton, and the remainder represented intermediate options.

The nine different strategies and the parish populations, broken down by age and sex, were read into the computer. The share of each parish

138

in the total number of out-patient attendances for the district was assumed to depend not only on the number of people living in the parish but also on the structure of the population. Elderly people are more likely than younger people to be out-patients, and women are more likely than men, so a parish with relatively large proportions of women and elderly people will probably produce more out-patients than a similar-sized parish with lower proportions in these groups. To take account of this effect, the population of each parish was weighted by multiplying the number of people in each age/sex category by the corresponding national hospital day and out-patient attendance rates, taken from the Report of the Resource Allocation Working Party (DHSS,1976). The age categories used were 0-4, 5-14, 15-44, 45-64, 65-74 and 75+ years.

In Chapter 3 it was estimated that at least 40% of out-patient attenances could be seen in viable decentralised clinics. A total of 33,000 attendances per year was used in the model, this being 40% of the 82,840 attendances in the district in 1975 (East Anglian Regional Health Authority, 1976). It may well be that future improvements in the service will cause the total to increase, but the overall level is of much less significance in the present exercise than the manner in which the total is distributed between clinics. In stage three, 33,000 annual attendances were distributed among the parishes according to the parish weightings established in stage two. This method assumes that out-patient attendances are not affected by distance, but are a function only of population size and structure.

For stage four, it was assumed that all out-patients considered suitable for community hospital clinics would attend the clinic nearest to their homes. This was recognised as an over-simplification of the likely situation but it was a necessary standardisation to ensure comparability between strategies. The more this condition is not met in reality, the more our results will underestimate the true travel distances and costs to the community. The nearest clinic was defined as the clinic with the shortest straight distance to the parish population centroid. Parish population centroids are map co-ordinates which represent the "centre of gravity" of the population of each parish and they are given in the small area statistics of the population census. The straight distance from each parish centroid to the nearest clinic under each strategy was calculated by applying Pythagoras' theorem to the map co-ordinates of centroids and clinics. This was taken to be the average distance of all the parish residents to that clinic. All distances within the towns of King's Lynn, Wisbech, Swaffham, Downham Market and Hunstanton were assumed to be 1.5 miles. For example, the residents of King's Lynn were assumed to live an average distance of 1.5 miles from the King's Lynn clinic. The figure of 1.5 miles was an arbitrary low distance made necessary by the fact that the "centroid distance" is an underestimate of average distance within the town itself. These measurements of distance were step five of the model.

The expected number of out-patient attendances calculated in stage three was not dependent on the distance of the parish to the clinic. Using the distances measured in stage five of the method, stage six went on to explore the alternative assumption, that short distances to an out-patient clinic encourage more trips and long distances tend to suppress trips. It will be recalled from Chapter 5 that there was some evidence of such an effect. As the results of the model are dependent upon the geographical origins of trips (and therefore must be sensitive to whether or not the distance effect is assumed to operate) it was decided to run two versions of the model : the first in which out-patient numbers were independent of distance and the second in which distance did affect numbers. In the second version the probability of attending a clinic from less than two miles was increased by multiplying the attendance estimates in that distance category by 1.67. Similarly, attendance estimates for parishes between two and ten miles from a clinic were multiplied by 1.08 and estimates for more distant parishes were decreased by multiplying them by 0.59. The adjustment coefficients originate from Table 5.7. Finally, to achieve comparability with the first version, the totals produced were scaled so that the strategy similar to the present situation (that is, clinics in King's Lynn and Wisbech) had exactly 33,000 out-patient attendances. For the other strategies the totals varied according to their accessibility levels. Once the revised expected numbers of out-patients per year from each parish under each strategy had been calculated, the program assigned them to their nearest clinic and calculated the distances travelled. In short, then, stage six consisted of a loop back through stages three, four and five with the assumption of trip suppression. From that point on, two sets of results were produced for each strategy : with and without the distance suppression effect.

In stage seven,the modal split in each parish (the proportions of out-patients using different forms of transport) was estimated from information about the level of car ownership in the parish, the distance of the parish from the clinic and the quality of the public transport service through the parish. Both the car ownership level (from the small area statistics of the 1971 census) and the public transport quality (either "good" with more than 15 buses per day or "bad" with less than that number) were read into the computer for each parish as pre-requisites for stage seven. Essentially, the method consisted of dividing the expected number of out-patients into car owning and non car owning groups according to the parish proportions and then allowing for the parish to clinic distance, as in Table 4.9. Slightly different versions of Table 4.9 were used according to whether the parish was comparatively well served or poorly served by public transport. The outcome was a breakdown of the expected out-patients in each parish into the proportions estimated to travel by ambulance or hospital car, by household car, by public transport, and on foot. The proportions varied from strategy to strategy as the distances to clinics altered.

The costs and times of the anticipated return journeys were then calculated in stage eight using the estimates of distance and mode of transport. For public transport users, the cost was estimated from the distance by applying the regression equation derived in Chapter 4. Costs for private car users were calculated on the basis of 6.618p per straight-line mile, which was also explained in Chapter 4. Costs for walkers and cyclists were assumed to be zero, and the costs of ambulances and hospital cars were not calculated, for want of information. Times were estimated for ambulance or hospital car users, for car users and for bus travellers from the equations given in Table 4.23. Walkers and cyclists were assigned the average time of 34 minutes in one direction, derived from the out-patients survey.

It will now be clear that the out-patients model was a complicated structure resting on many assumptions, some of which were uncertain or specific to the King's Lynn Health District. Its aim was to reproduce as closely as possible the distribution of out-patient trips expected to occur under different strategies of clinic location. Since all calculations were performed on a parish basis, the results were available parish by parish. To simplify the comparison of strategies, the parish results were aggregated to give totals or averages for the whole health district. These include the total distances and average distances travelled, the distances travelled by health service and non-health service transport, the total time spent on the trip and the total and average trip costs for those out-patients not travelling by health service transport. The results will be presented in the next section, after the characteristics of the in-patients and visitors model have been described.

In-patients and visitors model

The in-patients and visitors model was similar in many respects to the out-patients model. As in the out-patients method, estimation of the likely geographical origins of in-patients and visitors was followed by calculations concerning distance and cost. The basic stages were:

(1)   Establish the strategies of community hospital locations to be evaluated.

(2)   Calculate the expected share of each parish in the district's in-patients.

(3)   Estimate the expected number of in-patients per year from each parish.

(4)   Assign all in-patients to a community hospital, under each strategy.

(5)   Calculate the distances to be travelled by in-patients.

(6)   Estimate the modes of transport to be used by in-patients.

(7)   Estimate the trip costs of in-patients.

(8)   Estimate the number of visitors per year.

(9)   Allocate visitors' residences to parishes.

(10)   Calculate the distances to be travelled by visitors.

(11)   Estimate the modes of transport used by visitors.

(12)   Estimate the trip costs of visitors.

An important distinction was made in the model between preconvalescent, geriatric and elderly mentally infirm patients. These three groups were kept separate for the whole analysis. Four strategies for pre-convalescent patients, involving different combinations of community hospital facilities in King's Lynn, Wisbech, Swaffham and Downham Market, were tested. Another four strategies were tested for geriatric patients, and these involved different combinations of beds in King's Lynn, Wisbech, Swaffham and Hunstanton. For elderly mentally infirm patients only two strategies were investigated, the difference between them being whether or not accommodation for this group of patients was provided in Swaffham as well as in King's Lynn and Wisbech. Thus, the concept of a "community hospital" was left as flexible as possible, to include the three patient groups in any proportion. The strategies were selected in consultation with officers of the health authority, having regard to district bed norms and the hospital accommodation expected to be available in the 1980s. They are all thought to be real options, but they are not necessarily the options that will be considered by the Norfolk Area Health Authority. In other words, they were chosen for demonstration purposes only. Details of the strategies will be given in the results section.

Stage two of the model calculated each parish's share of the district's in-patients. As with out-patients, the number of in-patients produced by a parish was thought to be dependent not only on the population size of the parish but also on the age and sex composition of that population. Accordingly, the parish populations broken down by sex and age were taken from the 1971 census small area statistics and multiplied by the average number of beds used daily per million population for corresponding age/sex groups. The age groups were as in the out-patients model. For preconvalescent patients, the figures employed for average beds used daily per million population were those given for all departments excluding maternity. For geriatric and elderly mentally infirm patients, the separate geriatric figures were used. The source of these data was the Report on the Hospital In-patient Enquiry (DHSS, 1975).

In stage three, the total number of in-patients per year in each of the three patient categories was calculated by applying length of stay and bed occupancy rates to the number of beds. The bed numbers were those adopted as targets for a projected 1981 population by the Norfolk Area Health Authority (Norfolk Area Health Authority, 1978). For geriatric patients, the norm used was ten beds per thousand population over 65 years old, which gave 290 beds. For elderly mentally infirm patients, the norm of three beds per thousand population over 65 yielded 87 beds. The bed needs for preconvalescent patients was given as 81 beds, based on a norm of 0.5 beds per thousand population. The length of stay and bed occupancy figures used in the method were loosely based on district statistics (SH3 returns), with some adjustments to allow for likely trends. The statistics for preconvalescent patients were taken as 8.5 days average length of stay, with 90% bed occupancy. The corresponding figures for geriatric patients were 54.5 days average length of stay, with 75% occupancy. As elderly mentally infirm patients usually have long hospital stays, it was assumed that each bed would be occupied by the same person all year, so for them 87 beds was considered equivalent to 87 patients. The 290 geriatric beds were calculated as likely to be equivalent to 1457 geriatric patients per year on the basis of the bed occupancy and length of stay assumptions and similarly the 81 preconvalescent beds were calculated as accommodating 3130 patients per year. These patient totals were then divided among the parishes according to the shares established in the previous stage, to give an annual number of patients in each of the three categories for each parish.

A significant distinction between this model and the out-patients model was that whereas the latter allowed the size of each clinic to vary to accommodate however many out-patients there were living closest

to it, in this model the number of beds in any location was fixed.
As a result it was not always possible (although it was usually possible)
to allocate patients to the nearest community hospital, because the
nearest community hospital might be a particularly small unit whose beds
were already full. The rule adopted was to allocate patients in such a
way as to minimise the overall distance between homes and hospitals,
while making sure that every hospital unit would be working to capacity.
There is an accepted computer method for solving this type of problem
known as the transportation algorithm (Cooper, 1972), but as no strategy
involved more than three hospitals the catchment areas were delineated
by trial and error without the aid of the algorithm. The information
of which hospital each parish was to supply under each strategy was
then incorporated into the computer program for the model.

Step five employed the same assumptions for distance calculation as
in the out-patients model, that is, straight distances were measured
from hospitals to parish centroids and all distances within any of the
five towns were assumed to be 1.5 miles. In the in-patients model
there was the additional complication that preconvalescent patients were
expected to be transferred to the community hospital after a spell in
the district general hospital (or they might be staying in a community
hospital under observation before treatment at the district hospital).
Three distances were therefore measured for all preconvalescent patients
: from the home parish to the district general hospital in King's Lynn,
from the district general hospital to the community hospital and from
the community hospital to the home parish.

The method of estimating the proportions of in-patients being admitted
using different modes of transport (stage six) was cruder than the
method used in the out-patients model because less information was available. For preconvalescent and geriatric in-patients, the division into
transport modes was made entirely on the basis of distance travelled,
from Table 4.11. It was assumed that the proportions of patients
using the various modes of transport were the same for discharge as for
admission : an assumption that has not been tested. Preconvalescents'
journeys from the district general hospital to the community hospital
were assumed to be all by health service transport. No admission
information was available for elderly mentally infirm patients, so no
modes were estimated for this group. As the admission of elderly
mentally infirm patients is a comparatively rare event it was considered
unlikely that the costs incurred would influence hospital location
policy.

For stage seven the costs of round-trip travel for in-patients was
estimated as in the previous model, with the costs of public transport
calculated from equation 4.1 in Chapter 4, the costs of car travel as
6.618p per straight-line mile, no costs for walkers and no cost estimates for health service transport. No journey times were estimated
for in-patients, as the time of the admission and discharge journeys
was not considered to be a critical variable.

Stages 8-12 of the model are concerned with the visitors to hospital
patients. Since it was found in the surveys that each type of patient
generates its own distinctive visiting pattern, separate treatments of
visiting were made for the three categories of patient. In stage
eight, the annual numbers of visitors expected to be received by the

3130 preconvalescent patients, 1457 geriatric patients and 87 elderly
mentally infirm patients were calculated.   It has already been shown
that visiting rates to preconvalescent patients are dependent upon
length of stay and the distance from the hospital to the patient's
home (Table 5.21).   The average number of visitors per day for each
preconvalescent patient was calculated by applying equation 5.2.
For the purposes of this exercise, the influence of length of stay was
much less interesting than that of distance, so length of stay was held
constant at four days (that is, halfway between admission and average
discharge at 8.5 days).   The effect of the equation, then, was to vary
the number of visits expected by a patient according to the distance of
the patient's home from the hospital.   A patient living one mile away,
for example, was allocated 3.2 visits per day, a patient living six
miles away was given 2.3 visits per day, and patients from 15 and 25
miles away received 1.9 and 1.7 visits per day, respectively.   By
contrast, it will be recalled that geriatric patients' home distance had
virtually no effect on visiting rates.   Geriatric patients were assumed
to be halfway through their average stay of 54.5 days and when this halfway figure of 27 days was inserted into equation 5.1 a prediction of 1.2
visitor trips per day was produced for geriatric patients from any
distance.   Elderly mentally infirm patients (for whom no relationship
between visiting and length of stay or home distance was apparent) were
assigned their median number of two visits per month or 0.067 visits per
day.   Finally, the annual numbers of visitors anticipated for the three
categories of patient were derived by multiplying the average number of
visits one patient would expect in a day by the average length of stay
and by the number of patients in each category.   Preconvalescent
patients had a different total number of visitors under each strategy
as the distance decay effect was allowed to operate on different
configurations of hospitals.   No such effect was built into the geriatric
and elderly mentally infirm calculations so these categories each had the
same total of visitors under all strategies.

 Stage nine was possibly the most complex stage of the model.   Having
predicted the total number of visitors, the next task was to decide
where they were likely to have come from.   The estimate was made using
the information from Chapter 4 that 67% of visitors to preconvalescent
and geriatric patients and 56% of visitors to elderly mentally infirm
patients lived within two miles of the patient they were visiting.
These percentages were used to divide the visitors to every patient into
those who were estimated to live within two miles (who were allocated
to the same parish as the patient) and those estimated to live more than
two miles away.   The second group was spread randomly over the district
in proportion to the population of each parish or town, while still re-
taining a record of which patient and hospital each visitor was associated with.   The computer programe then found the annual total of
visitors allocated to each parish or town and kept a record of their
various hospital destinations.

Once the origins and destinations of visitors had been established,
the remaining stages 10-12 of the model were straightforward.   The
distances travelled were calculated precisely as before : that is, using
straight distances from parish centroids and distances of 1.5 miles
within towns.   The distances were then used to establish the modes of
transport of visitors, according to Table 4.17.   Visitors to elderly
mentally infirm patients were assumed to follow the same pattern of

modal split as the other categories of visitor.   The costs of car users for the return journey were then calculated at the rate of 6.618p per straight line mile and the costs incurred by bus users were estimated using equation 4.1.

Like the out-patients model, the in-patients and visitors model produced far more information than could readily be assimilated in order to compare planning strategies.   To simplify interpretation, the journeys of in-patients were grouped into those requiring health service transport and those which were on foot, by car or by bus (which collect-ively were termed "community transport").   All parish totals were added, to give results for the whole district.   The total miles travelled and the average journey distances were calculated for in-patients using either health service or community transport and for visitors.   Total and average costs were computed for all visitors and for the in-patients using community transport.

RESULTS AND STRATEGY EVALUATIONS

The four components of a community hospital that have been studied here - out-patient clinics and beds for preconvalescent, geriatric and elderly mentally infirm patients - have each been analysed under a series of locational options or strategies, but the strategies differ consider-ably between components.   Consequently, the four sets of results must be described separately.   The advantage of keeping the components separate in the evaluation stage is that the planner is enabled to build up a number of hospital units from the component parts so that their locations, sizes and patient-mixes may be tailored to fit local circum-stances.

Implications for out-patients

The locations of clinics considered in the nine strategies were as follows:

Strategy A : King's Lynn

Strategy B : King's Lynn, Wisbech

Strategy C : King's Lynn, Wisbech, Swaffham

Strategy D : King's Lynn, Wisbech, Downham

Strategy E : King's Lynn, Wisbech, Hunstanton

Strategy F : King's Lynn, Wisbech, Downham, Hunstanton

Strategy G : King's Lynn, Wisbech, Swaffham, Downham

Strategy H : King's Lynn, Wisbech, Swaffham, Hunstanton

Strategy I : King's Lynn, Wisbech, Swaffham, Downham, Hunstanton

The strategies with the catchment areas of the clinics are illustrated in Figure 6.1.

Table 6.1 shows that the numbers of out-patient attendances vary considerably from place to place and from one strategy to another.

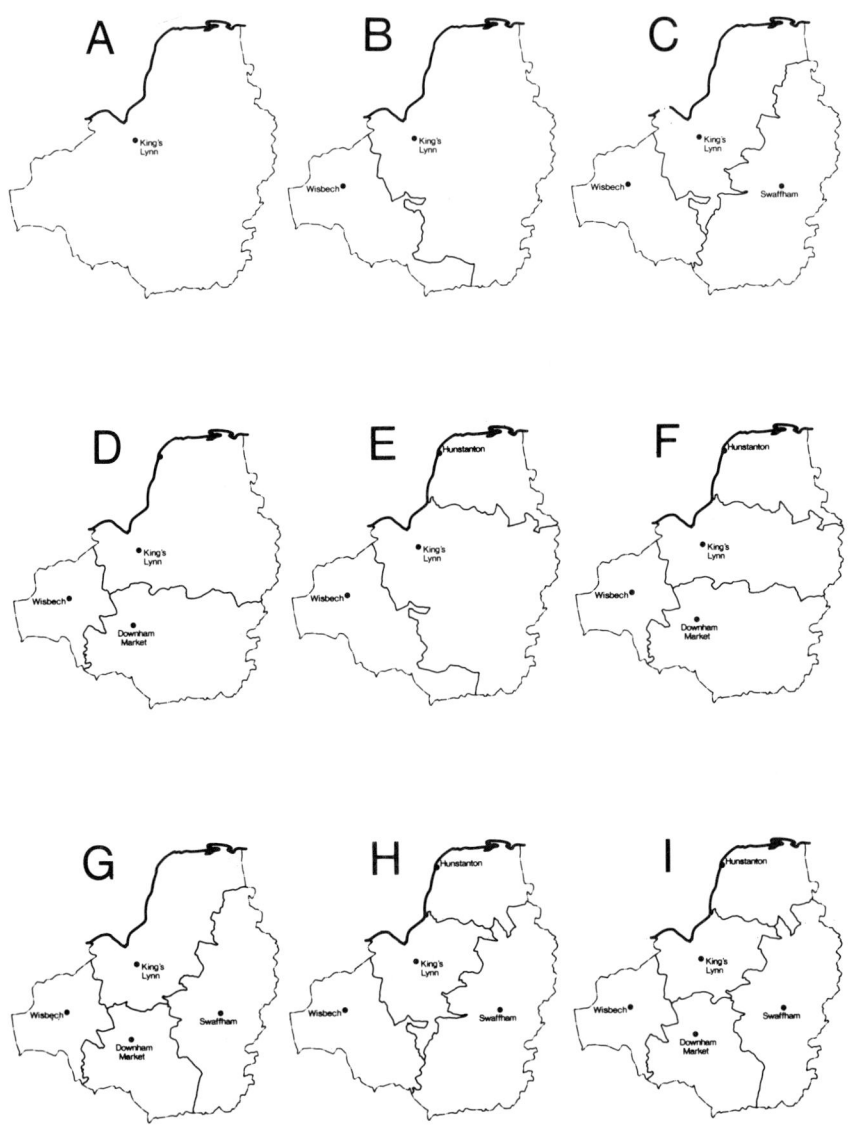

Figure 6.1 Strategies for out-patient clinics

146

For all strategies King's Lynn has the largest number, although the actual number King's Lynn would receive if all out-patients attended their nearest available clinic varies from 33,000 in strategy A to only 10,300 in strategy I. Of course, in addition to these, King's Lynn is assumed to receive the 60% of out-patients who must attend a district general hospital clinic. If King's Lynn is to share its "community hospital" clinics with Wisbech, strategy B shows that King's Lynn would receive approximately twice as many attendances as Wisbech.

Table 6.1
Out-patient attendances per year (in thousands) to each location

Strat -egy	King's Lynn	Wisbech	Swaffham	Downham	Hunstanton
A	33.0(28.0)	- -	- -	- -	- -
B	21.9(20.9)	11.4(12.1)	- -	- -	- -
C	15.1(16.5)	10.6(11.7)	7.5(6.8)	- -	- -
D	17.3(17.6)	8.1 (9.8)	- -	7.8(7.5)	- -
E	17.1(17.7)	11.4(12.1)	- -	- -	4.8(4.8)
F	12.5(14.4)	8.2 (9.8)	- -	7.8(7.5)	4.8(4.8)
G	14.3(15.7)	8.2 (9.8)	5.7(5.5)	5.0(5.6)	- -
H	11.1(13.8)	10.6(11.7)	7.4(6.7)	- -	4.2(4.4)
I	10.3(13.0)	8.2 (9.8)	5.6(5.4)	5.0(5.6)	4.2(4.4)

Note: Figures in brackets are under the assumption of suppression by distance.

Strategy I in Table 6.1 is particularly instructive as it gives the relative "drawing power" of the five towns if each town were the destination for out-patients living closest. King's Lynn followed by Wisbech clearly have the most populated catchment areas. The three smaller towns are able to attract markedly less trips. Of the three, Swaffham has the highest catchment population and Hunstanton the lowest. The relatively low catchment population of Hunstanton is emphasised in strategies C, D and E, which each posit the addition of one more location to clinics in King's Lynn and Wisbech. While both Swaffham and Downham Market would be expected to receive over 7,000 trips, Hunstanton is expected to attract considerably fewer. The superiority of Swaffham or Downham Market locations to Hunstanton is also shown in the remaining strategies F, G and H, which consider combinations of two locations additional to those in King's Lynn and Wisbech.

The conclusions reached above are based on the version of the model which does not take into account the suppression of out-patients' trips by increasing distance. The figures in brackets in Table 6.1 are expected attendances when the distance effect is taken into account. They show that although there are some differences in detail most of the observations made above remain valid. One exception to this is that Swaffham, unlike other locations receives fewer out-patient trips in all strategies than it did when trip suppression was not considered.

An implication of the trip suppression by distance assumption which deserves attention concerns the total number of attendances likely to

147

be made in each strategy.   If out-patient attendances to the present
clinics in King's Lynn and Wisbech really are the outcome of an inhibitory distance effect as was suggested in Chapter 5, then the dispersal
of clinics to more towns might be expected to "unlock" suppressed demand
and increase attendances.   Conversely, complete centralisation in King's
Lynn is expected to decrease the demand for clinic attendance.   Table
6.2 illustrates these effects by showing the attendances expected as a
percentage of those anticipated under strategy B (which comes closest
to the present situation).   If the distance effect measured in Chapter
5 is valid, then complete centralisation of out-patient clinics could
reduce demand to 85% of its present level.   Alternatively, complete
decentralisation of the clinics for which decentralisation is feasible
could increase demand by a further 16%.   This is an oversimplification,
of course, for in reality these increases or decreases in "demand" would
not be manifested in an obvious way.   Demand would quickly adjust to
the number of out-patient appointments available and the only measurable
effect would be a different geographical distribution of out-patient
origins.

Table 6.2
Out-patient attendances assuming suppression by distance

Strategy	Total attendances (thousands)	as % of B
A	28.0	85
B	33.0	100
C	35.0	106
D	34.9	106
E	34.5	105
F	36.4	110
G	36.6	111
H	36.6	111
I	38.2	116

Before considering the implications of the various strategies in
terms of travel distance and cost, it is worth noting that the modes
of transport used are not found to vary greatly between strategies
(Table 6.3).   Private transport (mostly by car) is dominant for all
strategies.   Otherwise the only feature of note is that the percentage
of trips by public transport and by NHS transport is greater for the
more concentrated strategies, whilst walking is more important for the
more dispersed strategies.   The assumption of trip suppression by
distance has little effect on the modal split.

A summary of the main results of the out-patients model (without the
assumption of trip suppression) is given in Table 6.4, where measures
relating to the 33,000 community hospital attendances appear together
with a breakdown into those travelling by health service transport
(ambulance and hospital car service) and those using "community
transport" (private cars, walking and public buses).

Table 6.3
Out-patients' mode of transport

Strategy	NHS	% of trips by each mode		
		Private	Public	Walking
A	15	65	13	6
B	13	66	11	10
C	12	67	10	11
D	12	66	10	11
E	12	67	10	11
F	11	67	10	12
G	11	67	9	12
H	11	67	9	12
I	11	68	9	13

Table 6.4
Out-patients model : summary of results

Strategies:	A	B	C	D	E	F	G	H	I
Out-patients	33.0	33.0	33.0	33.0	33.0	33.0	33.0	33.0	33.0
Mean dist.	9.9	7.4	5.8	6.2	6.4	5.2	5.0	4.8	4.1
Over 10 mls.	56	33	22	24	25	16	14	14	6
Total mls.	657	490	381	410	425	345	330	319	268
Total hours	34.9	29.4	25.5	26.6	27.1	24.4	23.8	23.4	21.7
NHS mls/pat.	23.2	18.5	14.8	16.0	16.5	13.7	13.3	12.3	9.8
NHS mls.	116	80	59	64	66	50	49	45	36
Comm.mls/pat.	19.1	14.1	11.0	11.8	12.3	9.9	9.5	9.2	7.8
Comm.mls.	541	410	322	346	359	295	281	274	232
Cost/pat.	1.05	.79	.63	.66	.69	.57	.54	.53	.45
Comm.cost	35.1	26.4	20.9	22.1	23.1	18.9	18.1	17.7	15.0

KEY Out-patients: Number of out-patient attendances per year (thousands)
Mean dist: Mean distance from clinic (miles)
Over 10 mls: Percentage attendances over 10 miles from clinic
Total mls: Total patient miles per year (thousands)
Total hours: Total travel time per year (thousand hours)
NHS mls/pat: Health service transport mean miles per patient
NHS mls: Health service transport total patient miles per year (thousands)
Comm.mls/pat: Community transport mean miles per patient
Comm.mls: Community transport total patient miles per year (thousands)
Cost/pat: Community transport mean cost per patient (£)
Comm.cost: Community transport total cost per year (£ thousands)

As the number of locations increases it is to be expected that average trip lengths will fall. This effect is clearly demonstrated in Table 6.4. It shows that when there are five locations (strategy I) average distances to the clinic and total travel distances are predicted to be less than half what they would be with a single location (strategy A). This suggests that a policy of dispersing clinics might be extremely effective in reducing trip lengths. However, the results also suggest that there are likely to be practical limits to the process. This is because each additional location produces a progressively smaller reduction in trip lengths. The addition of out-patient clinics at Wisbech to existing ones at King's Lynn produces the largest reduction in trip lengths. The effects of adding a third location are smaller, as are the effects of a fourth and fifth location.

The same is also true of the prospects for reducing the number of long trips (defined as those over 10 miles). These can be greatly reduced by an increase in the number of locations but the effects of additional locations becomes progressively less.

The trip length measures may be examined to find out which of the three locations in smaller towns produces the greatest reductions. At the stage of the addition of a third location (strategies C, D and E) the results suggest that Swaffham performs best, in terms of both the lowest mean trip lengths and the smallest number of long trips. Hunstanton is the least effective. At the next stage (strategies F, G and H) it is the combination of Swaffham and Hunstanton (strategy H) that performs best. However, it should be noted that there is little to choose on this count between this and strategy G, the combination of Swaffham and Downham Market.

All the conclusions drawn on the basis of the total journey miles or the average distances from the nearest clinic apply also to the differences in total travel time between strategies, except that the travel time saved by a policy of dispersed clinics is proportionately less than the reduction in travel distance. This is for two main reasons. Firstly, as the number of locations increases, the number of out-patients walking to clinics also increases, and walking tends to be slower than other modes. Secondly, no matter how long the journey is, the extra time taken waiting for a bus or parking a car is likely to be the same. However, Table 6.4 includes time estimates only for the out-patients themselves and not for the people accompanying them. The inclusion of companions' times would tend to increase the difference between concentrated and dispersed strategies.

The next information in Table 6.4 relates to the journeys expected to be made by health service transport in transporting out-patients to and from clinics (but not including the initial and terminal trips from and to the vehicle's base). A topic of considerable importance when planning the location of clinics is what demands are likely to be placed on the ambulance service and on the hospital car service. Would a more dispersed pattern of clinics produce savings in these aspects of NHS transport by reducing the numbers or lengths of trips they are required to undertake? Table 6.4 suggests that there is indeed considerable scope for reducing the patient miles carried by NHS transport. With five locations total patient miles would be less than a third what they would be with a single location in King's Lynn.

Assuming that costs are related to mileage it is therefore likely that savings in NHS ambulance and car service costs would result from a dispersal of out-patient clinics. As we have been unable to acquire realistic figures on the costs per patient mile of either the hospital car service or the ambulance service it has not been possible to give an estimate of the NHS transport costs. When the costs per patient mile become known, total costs may be estimated from the information in Table 6.4 by a simple multiplication. Taking patient miles as a guide to costs, it appears that as the number of dispersed clinics increases, NHS transport costs are expected to decrease, although the amount of decrease is less at each step. The strategy with three clinics at King's Lynn, Wisbech and Swaffham involves only half the patient miles of strategy A and appears particularly efficient.

For the patients who make their own way to the clinic by car, by bus or on foot, similar conclusions may be drawn. The average return trip distance is reduced from 19.1 miles to 7.8 miles from strategy A to strategy I. Of the three-location strategies C appears to be the best, and of the four-location choices H seems preferable.

The costs of private and public transport for one return trip are expected to average £1.05 for strategy A, ranging down to a low 45p for strategy I. Average costs are, of course, a poor measure of hardship in particular cases, but on the average decentralisation of clinics can cut average community travel costs in half. Also of interest are the total transport costs expected to be incurred by the community. These vary between £35,000 and £15,000 per year from strategy A to strategy I. It has already been emphasised that such estimates are no better than the collection of assumptions that have produced them, but they do indicate the order of magnitude of the costs involved. The community cost estimates can now be weighed in the balance against the health service costs incurred by decentralisation of clinics : the costs of consultants' time and travel, the costs of maintaining extra buildings and extra ancillary staff, and so on. If community transport costs may be reduced from £35,000 to £21,000 by establishing extra clinics in Wisbech and Swaffham and to £18,000 by adding one more in Hunstanton (and if health service transport costs may be reduced proportionately), then where is the best balance struck? Information such as that in Table 6.4 will enable such decisions to be made on rational grounds, with the assumptions laid bare.

So far, the results have been presented as if distance has no discouraging effect on out-patient attendances. If such an effect does operate (and in the manner hypothesised in Chapter 5) then the effects of the strategies might be as in Table 6.5. Because it encourages shorter trips at the expense of longer trips, the suppression assumption yields considerably reduced average distances per patient and costs per patient. The total miles, hours or costs are usually decreased by the application of the assumption, but not necessarily so because (with all other things being equal) the number of attendances is increased as the clinics are made more dispersed. In general, however, the strategies retain their relative positions under the suppression assumption. As the number of locations increases, all the indices of distance, time and cost are reduced. Of the three-location strategies, C is still superior on all indices, while there is now little to choose between G and H of the four-location strategies. One difference between this table and Table 6.4, though, is in the much smaller distinction in times and costs across the strategies in Table 6.5. The reason for this phenomenon is that the increased number of shorter trips in Table 6.5 all involve "terminal" times and costs : that is, times and costs incurred whatever the distance. It is these terminal costs together with the greater number of trips that increase the totals for the more dispersed strategies. If the trip suppression assumption is true, then decentralisation would produce much less savings in community costs than Table 6.4 suggested, although it would, of course, produce the benefits of more out-patient attendances.

Table 6.5

Outpatients model : results under the assumption of suppression by distance

Strategies:	A	B	C	D	E	F	G	H	I
Out-patients	28.0	33.0	35.0	34.9	34.5	36.4	36.6	36.6	38.2
Mean dist.	7.8	5.6	4.6	4.7	4.9	4.2	4.0	4.0	3.5
Over 10 mls.	38	19	12	13	14	8	7	7	3
Total mls.	438	368	320	331	339	304	295	293	268
Total hours	25.9	25.7	24.7	25.1	25.3	24.8	24.6	24.4	24.2
NHS mls/pat.	17.4	12.9	11.0	11.5	11.8	10.2	9.9	9.7	8.1
NHS mls.	73	56	46	48	49	41	40	39	34
Comm.mls/pat.	15.3	10.8	8.9	9.2	9.6	8.1	7.8	7.8	6.9
Comm.mls.	365	312	274	283	290	263	255	254	234
Cost/pat.	.80	.57	.48	.49	.51	.44	.42	.43	.37
Comm.cost	22.3	19.0	16.8	17.1	17.7	15.9	15.5	15.6	14.3

KEY	Out-patients:	Number of out-patient attendances per year (thousands)
	Mean dist:	Mean distance from clinic (miles)
	Over 10 mls:	Percentage attendances over 10 miles from clinic
	Total mls:	Total patient miles per year (thousands)
	Total hours:	Total travel time per year (thousand hours)
	NHS mls/pat:	Health Service transport mean miles per patient
	NHS mls:	Health Service transport total patient miles per year (thousands)
	Comm.mls/pat:	Community transport mean miles per patient
	Comm.mls:	Community transport total patient miles per year (thousands)
	Cost/pat:	Community transport mean cost per patient (£)
	Comm.cost:	Community transport total cost per year (£ thousands)

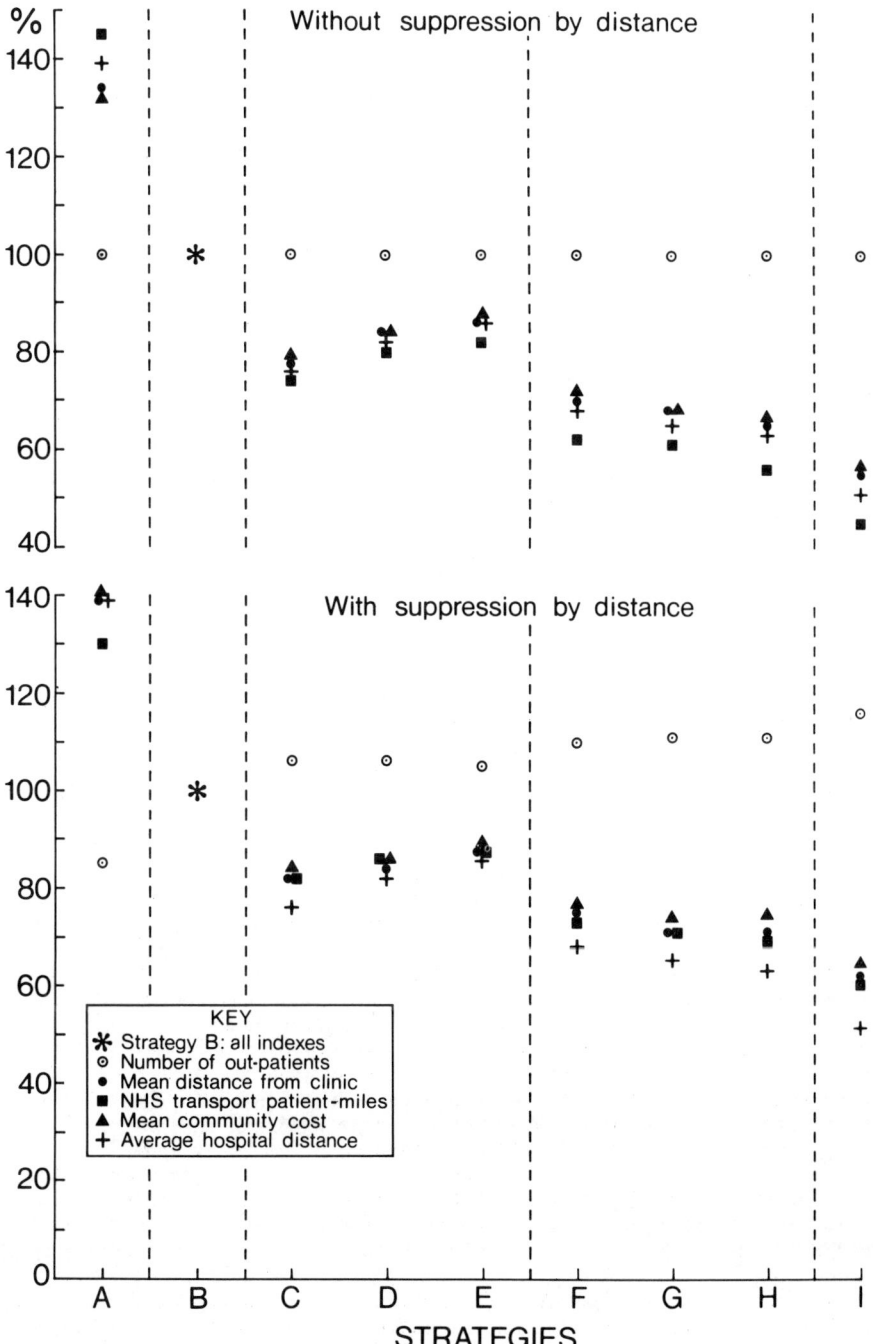

Figure 6.2   Implications of out-patient strategies

A selection of results from the model is shown in Figure 6.2. Results are given both without and with the trip suppression assumption. Indices for all strategies are expressed as percentages of the same measures for strategy B, the option with clinics in King's Lynn and Wisbech which represents the existing situation.

The figure shows, for example, that centralisation of all clinics in King's Lynn (strategy A) would increase the mean distance to 134% of its level at the present time, while devolution to five clinic centres would reduce the mean distance to 55% its current value. If the trip suppression assumption is applied, the corresponding figures are 139% and 62%. Similarly, any strategy may be compared with strategy B on any index, by reading the appropriate percentage from the graph. Considering all indices together, the pattern of symbols gives a visual impression of the relative differences between the strategies. The increase in accessibility as more clinics are added, from strategy A to strategy I, is evident from the graph. What is also clear from a comparison of the upper and lower parts of the diagram is that the trip suppression assumption produces slightly smaller relative differences between the strategies than the model without the assumption. The relative performances of the strategies, however, are identical whether the suppression assumption is applied or not. The same is true of the different indices used: they all produce precisely the same order of strategies (with the slight exception of identical measures for suppressed strategies G and H).

In order of decreasing accessibility the strategies are ranked : I, H, G, F, C, D, E, B and A. If a third clinic location were to be added to King's Lynn and Wisbech, Swaffham would be the most advantageous. The most efficient system of four clinics would be King's Lynn, Wisbech, Swaffham and Hunstanton.

Implications for preconvalescent patients and their visitors.

Table 6.6 shows how the proposed 81 preconvalescent beds for the King's Lynn Health District were divided between towns in the four strategies tested. Strategy J is meant to represent the situation when the new district general hospital is in service and all preconvalescent patients are transferred to Wisbech, Swaffham and Downham Market. This arrangement is not expected to be permanent as Stow Hall near Downham Market is not owned by the Norfolk Area Health Authority and is likely to be relinquished in the long term. The remaining three strategies, therefore, are different ways of redistributing Stow Hall's 40 preconvalescent beds. In strategy K they are accommodated in one of the Wisbech hospitals. In strategy L they go to King's Lynn and in strategy M King's Lynn takes 29 and Swaffham Cottage Hospital is extended to accommodate the remaining 11. The catchment areas of the preconvalescent units (assuming patients are assigned as much as possible to the unit nearest their home) are illustrated for each strategy in Figure 6.3.

All four strategies examined for preconvalescent patients incorporate either two or three hospital units, unlike the out-patient strategies which covered a wider range from one to five clinic locations. The differences between the four preconvalescent strategies in terms of transport and accessibility implications are therefore much less than the differences observed for the out-patient options.   Table 6.7 summarises the results from the preconvalescent model.

Table 6.6
Number of preconvalescent beds in each location for strategies J - M

Location	J	K	L	M
King's Lynn			40	29
Wisbech	23	63	23	23
Swaffham	18	18	18	29
Downham Market	40			

The four preconvalescent strategies accommodate the same number of patients (3,130 per year) in different combinations of hospital locations.   When the straight distance from the patient's home to the hospital is estimated, strategy L, with an average of 6.0 miles, appears considerably more advantageous than strategy K, whose average is 10.2 miles.   Strategy M. is very close to L, and J occupies an intermediate position.   The same is true when the measure used is the percentage of patients estimated to live more than ten miles from their preconvalescent unit.   However, these measures do not take account of the fact that most preconvalescent patients will be either on their way to, or back from, the district general hospital in King's Lynn.

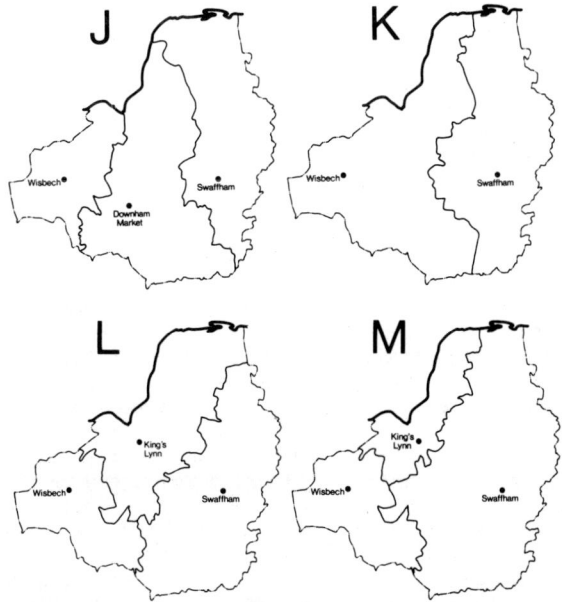

Figure 6.3   Strategies for preconvalescent patients

When the total patient miles from home to home via both the district
general hospital and the nearest community hospital are estimated, the
relative differences between strategies are slightly reduced, but the
ordering remains the same. Strategy K is the least efficient, with
approximately 102,500 patient miles per year and strategy L the most,
with 72,800 patient miles per year.

Table 6.7
Preconvalescent model : summary of results

Strategies:	J	K	L	M
Patients				
Number of patients per year (thousands)	3.13	3.13	3.13	3.13
Mean distance from hospital (mls)	8.6	10.2	6.0	6.5
Percentage over 10 miles from hospital	43	54	23	28
Total patient miles per year (thousands)	94.9	102.5	72.8	79.9
Health Service transport:				
Mean miles per patient (home-DGH)	10.6	10.6	10.6	10.6
Mean miles per patient (DGH-CH)	11.7	12.5	7.2	9.0
Mean miles per patient (CH-home)	9.2	10.9	6.4	7.0
Total patient miles per year (thousands)	85.2	92.4	63.7	70.8
Community transport:				
Mean miles per patient	14.3	15.6	12.2	12.6
Total patient miles per year (thousands)	9.7	10.1	9.0	9.1
Mean cost per patient (£)	.82	.95	.66	.69
Total cost per year (£ thousands)	.60	.63	.56	.56
Visitors				
Number of visitors per year (thousands)	61.6	59.4	66.2	65.5
Mean distance from hospital (mls)	9.3	10.6	7.4	7.9
Percentage over 10 miles from hospital	48	55	34	38
Total visitor miles per year (millions)	1.15	1.26	0.98	1.04
Mean cost per visitor (£)	.57	.65	.44	.48
Total cost per year (£ thousands)	35.0	38.5	29.2	31.1

Preconvalescent patients are expected to be expensive for the
ambulance service because of the extra trip between the general hospital
and the community hospital. For the patients estimated to be travelling by health service transport (and this includes all patients for
transfer between hospitals) the average distances per patient for each
section of the journey are separated in the table. The location of
community hospitals naturally has no effect on the distance from patients'
home to the general hospital. While strategies J and K have community
hospitals which are further on average from patients' homes than
strategies L and M, the factor that accentuates the difference between
the two pairs of strategies is the lack of preconvalescent services in
King's Lynn in J and K. This has the effect of inflating the average
distance between the general hospital and community hospitals compared
with L and M. In terms of the implications for the ambulance service

there is consequently a large gap between the first two and the last
two options. While strategy K would involve some 92,400 patient miles
per year, the corresponding figure for L is only 63,700. To the extent
that ambulance costs are proportional to patient miles, the opening of a
40 bed preconvalescent unit in King's Lynn rather than in Wisbech is
expected to reduce ambulance running costs by almost one-third.

In comparison to the ambulance costs, the total transport costs for
preconvalescent patients who pay for their own journey are expected to
be extremely low. The model predicts total annual community costs
varying from £630 in strategy K to £560 in strategies L and M. For the
individual patients expected to travel mostly by car, average cost
estimates vary from 66p to 95p for the double journey.

In the lower section of Table 6.7 the implications for visitors are
summarised. The only measure in the table for which high values
denote greater efficiency and low values represent lesser efficiency is
that of the number of visitors per year. Because of the inhibitory
effect of distance on visiting rates, the strategy with the most accessible combination of preconvalescent units (L) is expected to attract
about 11% more visitors than the least accessible option (K), about 7%
more than strategy J and only 1% more than M. The ability to generate
more visiting trips and thereby avoid the social costs of some suppressed visiting demand counts in favour of strategies L and M.

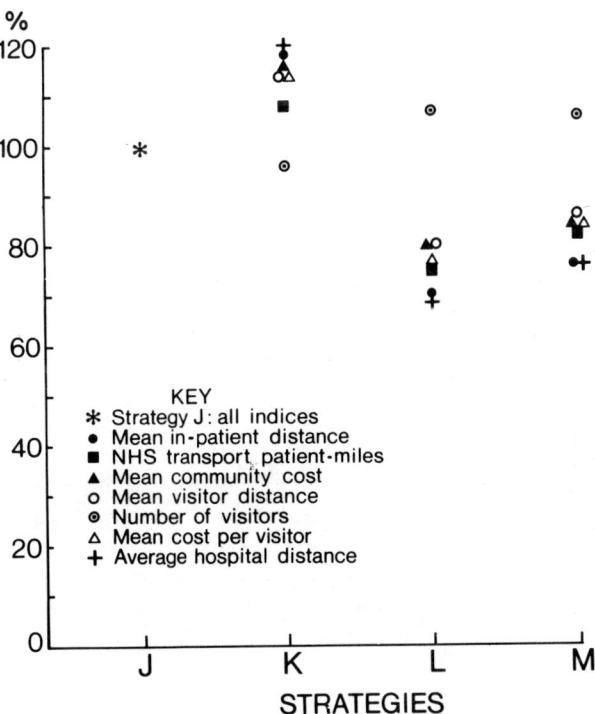

Figure 6.4   Implications for preconvalescent patients

All the distance and cost measures for visitors confirm the positions of the strategies established by the other indices in the table, with L closely followed by M being the most efficient, K the least and J occupying an intermediate position. It is interesting to compare the order of magnitude of the predicted visitors' total miles travelled with the patient miles for health service transport. Visitors are expected to cover considerably more distance than health service transport for admissions, transfers and discharges; in fact, 13-15 times more, depending on the strategy. This travel by visitors is estimated to cost the community between £29,200 and £38,500 per year, again according to strategy. It is worth emphasising that these sums of expenditure are generated by only 81 hospital beds.

A selection of relevant indices is used to convey a visual comparison between the four preconvalescent strategies in Figure 6.4. All indices are expressed as percentages of their value in strategy J, the likely situation when the district general hospital is working. The distance and cost indices of strategy K are 105-118% of those for strategy J, while the measures for strategies L and M are 70-93% and 76-93% respectively of J's values. Clearly, from the point of view of accessibility for patients, visitors and health service transport, options L and M with additional preconvalescent accommodation in King's Lynn are much preferable to the Wisbech-Swaffham solution. A 40 bed unit in King's Lynn would be more accessible and convenient than 29 beds in King's Lynn and an extra 11 beds in Swaffham, but only marginally so.

Implications for geriatric patients and their visitors

Based on the projected 1981 population figures, 290 beds are expected to be needed for geriatric patients in the King's Lynn Health District. Of these, about 86 beds will be for assessment and rehabilitation, accommodated in the district general hospital. The West Norfolk and King's Lynn Hospital is expected to be able to accommodate 100 geriatric beds and one or other of the Wisbech hospitals a further 50 beds. Thus, it appears possible that in the early 1980s King's Lynn will have about 186 geriatric beds and Wisbech about 50. To take the total of geriatric beds to the norm of 290 requires a further 54 beds. It is the location of these remaining 54 beds that is the variable element in the four geriatric strategies examined. Details are given in Table 6.8. Strategy N postulates the extra beds being provided in the town of King's Lynn, perhaps in the district general hospital or perhaps in another unit. Strategy O assumes they are provided in Swaffham, an option that would require building and a substantial increase in Swaffham's hospital population. In strategy P, the 54 beds are assigned to Wisbech, and in strategy Q to Hunstanton. The last strategy would again require a new unit, since the present hospital in Hunstanton is not suitable for geriatric patients. The catchment areas of the geriatric units of all strategies (assuming patients are assigned as much as possible to their nearest unit) are illustrated in Figure 6.5

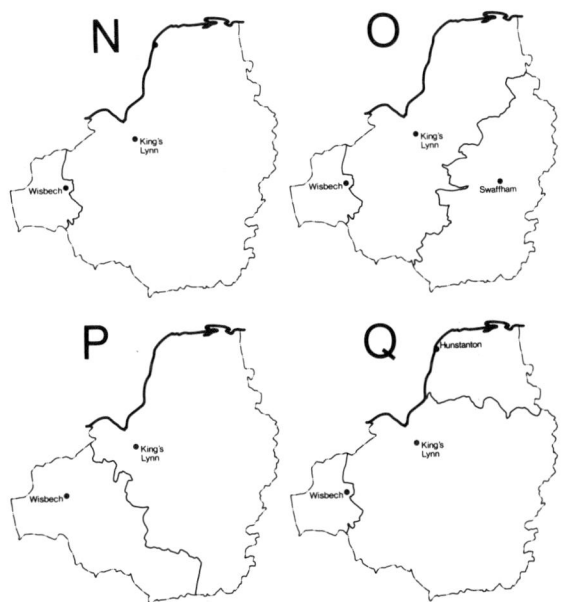

Figure 6.5   Strategies for geriatric patients

Table 6.8

Number of geriatric beds in each location for strategies N-Q

Location:	N	O	P	Q
King's Lynn	240	186	186	186
Wisbech	50	50	104	50
Swaffham		54		
Hunstanton				54

Although the number of geriatric beds assigned is three and a half times the number of preconvalescent beds in the district, the number of geriatric patients is reduced to less than half the number of preconvalescent patients because of their longer stays.   About 1,460 geriatric patients per year are anticipated (Table 6.9).   They are expected to travel between 19,800 and 24,500 miles, according to strategy.   These totals and the average distances per patient are much reduced from the corresponding preconvalescent figures because the latter included the general hospital to community hospital transfer and the long home to general hospital trip, as well as omitting the favourable King's Lynn location in two options.   Ambulance transport miles (and consequently costs) are also much reduced for geriatric patients : to between 14 and 18 miles per patient and annual totals of 15,900 - 20,300 patient miles. The total costs incurred by the small number of geriatric patients or their relatives expected to provide their own transport are a mere £240-£260 per annum.

Table 6.9
Geriatric model : summary of results

Strategies:	N	O	P	Q
Patients				
Number of patients per year (thousands)	1.46	1.46	1.46	1.46
Mean distance from hospital (mls)	8.4	6.8	7.8	7.0
Percentage over 10 miles from hospital	44	32	38	31
Total patient miles per year (thousands)	24.5	19.8	22.8	20.3
Health Service transport:				
Mean miles per patient	18.1	14.6	16.9	15.1
Total patient miles per year (thousands)	20.3	15.9	18.7	16.4
Community transport:				
Mean miles per patient	12.5	10.6	11.7	10.5
Total patient miles per year (thousands)	4.2	3.9	4.1	3.9
Mean cost per patient (£)	.76	.65	.71	.64
Total cost per year (£ thousands)	.26	.24	.25	.24
Visitors				
Number of visitors per year (thousands)	94.6	94.6	94.6	94.6
Mean distance from hospital (mls)	9.0	8.3	8.8	8.6
Percentage over 10 miles from hospital	48	42	46	42
Total visitor miles per year (millions)	1.70	1.57	1.67	1.62
Mean cost per visitor (£)	.54	.50	.53	.52
Total cost per year (£ thousands)	51.2	47.1	50.3	48.9

The implications for geriatric patients suggested in Table 6.9 differ
less between strategies than was the case with preconvalescent strategies.
For only two of the nine indices used does the most efficient strategy
drop below 80% of the measure for the least efficient strategy.   These
are for the percentage of patients living more than ten miles from a
hospital (this index in strategy Q is 70% its value in strategy N) and
the total health service patient miles per year, where strategy O is
78% of the value of strategy N.   All the other measures indicate a
similarity greater than 80% between the most accessible and the least
accessible strategies.   The least accessible strategy according to all
the indices of patient transport is N.   This is the option where over
four-fifths of the beds are in King's Lynn and the remainder are in
Wisbech.   The second most inaccessible is P, in which the division of
beds is almost two-thirds in King's Lynn and slightly more than one
third in Wisbech.   The strategies incorporating a third hospital
location, in Swaffham and Hunstanton for O and Q respectively, are the
most efficient for patient transport.   Most, but not all, indices
give the Swaffham strategy a very slight advantage over the Hunstanton
option.

These conclusions are reinforced by the indices of visitor transport.
All strategies produce the same estimated number of visitors per year
as, it will be recalled, no inhibitory effect of distance could be shown
for visitors to geriatric patients.   The other measures give the

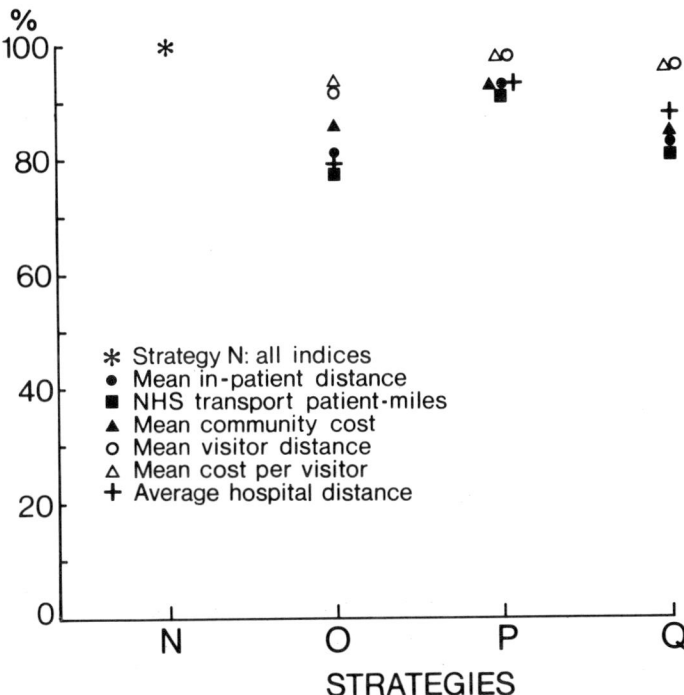

Figure 6.6   Implications for geriatric patients

options in decreasing order of accessibility as: O, Q, P and N.   The
figures for total visitor miles per year also make it clear that the
distances travelled by visitors vastly outweigh the distances covered
by ambulances for geriatric admissions and discharges.   The total
visitor distances are predicted by the model as being 84-99 times
greater than total health service patient-miles, depending on the
strategy.   While average costs to visitors are low, the total annual
costs of visiting patients occupying 290 geriatric beds are estimated
as varying between £47,100 in strategy O to £51,200 in strategy N.

Figure 6.6 is a summary diagram to illustrate the relative positions
of a small selection of indices for the geriatric strategies.   The
cross symbol, representing the measure of "average hospital distance"
will be referred to later.

Implications for visitors to elderly mentally infirm patients

Only two hospital strategies for elderly mentally infirm patients were
tested.   The King's Lynn Health District at present has no provision
for elderly mentally infirm patients, although 87 beds are calculated
as being needed on the basis of its 1981 population.   Strategy R
postulates a unit of 20 beds (thought to be about the minimum viable
size) in Wisbech and the remaining 67 beds in King's Lynn.   Strategy
S includes a unit of 20 beds in Swaffham as well as 20 beds in Wisbech
and 47 in King's Lynn.   The catchment areas of the two strategies are
shown in Figure 6.7.   By comparing the results of R and S, it ought
to be possible to gauge the benefits of a separate small unit in
Swaffham.

161

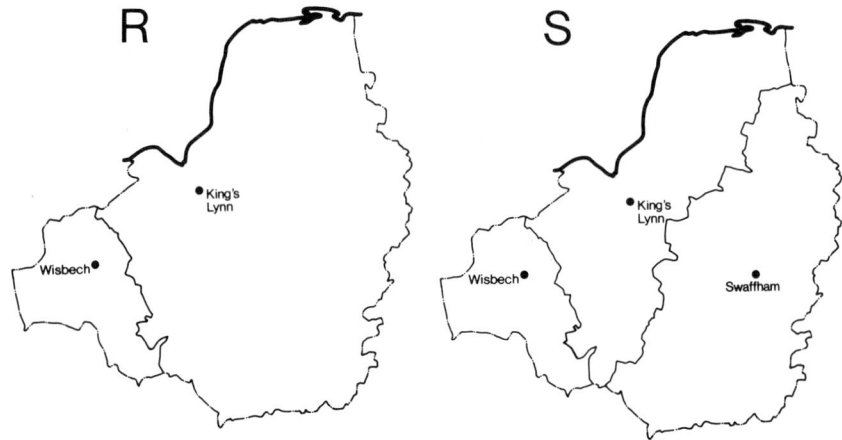

Figure 6.7   Strategies for elderly mentally infirm patients

Because of the extensive lengths of stay of elderly mentally infirm patients and the relatively small number of beds involved, the costs of transporting patients are expected to be minor and unlikely to influence hospital location policy.   We therefore concentrate on the distances and costs of visitors to elderly mentally infirm patients.

Estimates are given to Table 6.10.   The most striking feature of the table, compared with those for the other two types of patient, is the small number of visitors anticipated.   The 87 patients are together expected to receive approximately 2,100 visitors per year, at a cost to the visitors of about £1,150 in strategy R and £1,110 in strategy S. Not only are overall visiting costs low but also the differences between strategies is minimal.   Low total costs, of course, obscure the fact that some visitors may have high costs, but the other measures in the table suggest that the number of visitors with high costs are unlikely to be much reduced by opening a new unit at Swaffham.   The percentage of visitors expected to live more than ten miles from hospital is only improved from 48% to 43% in strategy S.

Table 6.10
Elderly mentally infirm model : summary of results

Strategies:	R	S
Visitors		
Number of visitors per year (thousands)	2.1	2.1
Mean distance from hospital (mls)	9.0	8.7
Percentage over 10 miles from hospital	48	43
Total visitor miles per year (thousands)	38.2	36.8
Mean cost per visitor (£)	.54	.52
Total cost per year (£ thousands)	1.15	1.11

Comparison of the other indices between the two strategies shows that S is superior to R generally only to the extent of a three or four percent difference. Spreading the future provision for elderly mentally infirm patients to Swaffham as well as King's Lynn and Wisbech cannot be said to increase appreciably the accessibility for visitors.

A SIMPLER EVALUATION METHOD

The results of the evaluation models presented above are the best estimates we can make with the information available of the implications of the planning strategies for patients' and visitors' travel. It is as well to remember that the simple numbers appearing in the tables are the product of several assumptions and many stages of calculation. In the out-patients model, over a hundred operations were performed by the computer for every parish in each strategy, and more than two hundred different operations were required for the in-patients and visitors model. Altogether, well over half a million calculations were necessary to produce the tables of results in this chapter. Even allowing for the fact that a human can take some short cuts not available to a computer, the task is clearly beyond the capacity of a willing planning assistant equipped with a desk calculator! A computer is necessary for this type of modelling and developing the required programs could be expected to take a matter of months, not days. In short, the method is a cumbersome one, unlikely to be widely applied unless a simple approximation can be found.

It has already been noted that all the different indices used produced the same relative ordering of strategies. There were only a few minor exceptions to this rule. To be acceptable, any approximation must be capable of reproducing the ranking of strategies and measuring their relative efficiencies. Although it is interesting to have an estimate of the total cost to the community or the total patient-miles transported by ambulance, for example, the absolute values of any of the indices used are much less significant for policy decisions than the variations in values between strategies. In any case, relative differences can be measured much more confidently than absolute levels.

For the models reported here, the absolute values of the results are known to be imprecise. The town and parish populations on which the whole evaluation is based, for example, are from the 1971 census whereas the strategies tested are options for the 1980s. We could, of course, have used 1981 or 1986 population projections for the exercise but simple projections would merely have increased or decreased the total number of people (and population forecasts are not notably reliable) without changing the age and sex composition at the parish level. On balance, it seemed better to use solid 1971 population information rather than crude estimates of 1981 totals in conjunction with 1971 age/sex break-downs. In the out-patients model, the number of out-patients consider-ed was based on 40% of the 1975 King's Lynn District total. Again, a projection of out-patient numbers in the district to 1981 or some other date could be made (with the inevitable chance of error), but then our estimate of 40% would still remain no more than an estimate. One solution would be to run the model with several different percentages of several different projections, but the absurdly large volume of results produced would differ only in absolute terms and not at all in relative terms.

In the in-patient model, the absolute numbers of patients depend on the number of beds notionally assigned, together with the length of stay and bed occupancy characteristics of the patients. An error in any one of the estimates used would produce different numbers of patients and consequently different numbers of visitors, different amounts of expenditure, and so on. It would not, however, alter the relative rankings of the strategies. All the models relied heavily on the proportions of people using different modes of transport found in surveys conducted in 1977. Needless to say, with car ownership increasing in the district these figures are in a state of flux and are expected to change the absolute values of the indices used by the 1980s. As a final example, the cost estimates made in the model are already out of date, because they are based on 1977 figures. They could certainly be made to appear more realistic, by incorporating an estimate of inflation between 1977 and 1981, but for what purpose? All these refinements involve further assumptions, only one of which needs to be inaccurate before the edifice tumbles. The point is that it is extremely difficult to forecast the absolute values of any index and extra effort is soon met by diminishing returns. The relative values between strategies, on the other hand, depend on far fewer assumptions and appear to be comparatively stable.

A straightforward measure that can be used to gauge the relative levels of accessibility of different hospital location strategies is the "average hospital distance". This is simply the average distance of all members of the population to the nearest appropriate hospital. When hospital catchments have been drawn, the average hospital distance is calculated by multiplying the population of each parish or town by the distance to hospital, adding the products for all parishes and towns in the district and then dividing by the district's total population. Using the conventions of straight distances measured from parish centroids and distances of 1.5 miles within towns, the average hospital distances were calculated for all the strategies examined. The results appear in Table 6.11

Table 6.11
Average hospital distances for all strategies (miles)

Out-patient strategies:

A	B	C	D	E	F	G	H	I
9.6	6.9	5.3	5.7	5.9	4.7	4.5	4.3	3.5

In-patient strategies:

J	K	L	M	N	O	P	Q	R	S
8.3	9.9	5.7	6.3	8.0	6.3	7.4	7.0	7.5	5.9

When the average hospital distances based on the whole population are compared with the mean out-patient and in-patient distances, the average hospital distances are almost invariably shorter, sometimes by as much as half a mile. This is due to the population distribution in the study district, where elderly people make up a greater proportion of the population away from the towns than they do close to the towns. Because elderly people are more likely to be hospital patients than

164

younger people, the average patient's distance to hospital is greater than the average person's distance. The two measures, however, do place the strategies in the same order of relative efficiency. They would only fail to do this in a situation where the age and sex composition of the population varied markedly from one part of the study area to another.

Comparison of the average hospital distances with the other indices used is facilitated by taking one strategy as a benchmark and expressing the others relative to it. This has already been done for the other indices in Figures 6.2, 6.4 and 6.6. For the out-patient strategies, Figure 6.2 shows that the average hospital distance is an excellent summary of the relative levels of mean patient distances from clinics, health service transport patient miles and mean community transport costs. When the longer out-patient trips are suppressed and the shorter journeys encouraged, the average hospital distance not surprisingly exaggerates the differences between strategies, but still preserves the order. Similar patterns are observable for the pre-convalescent and geriatric strategies in Figures 6.4 and 6.6. Average hospital distance is generally a good approximation to the relative levels of the mean distance, health service distance and mean cost for patients but it tends to exaggerate the differences in distance and cost for visitors. Perhaps the visitor measures varied less than the in-patient measures because the fact that one third of visitors (44% for visitors to elderly mentally infirm patients) were spread over the entire district ensured a proportion of relatively long journeys whatever the strategy. Certainly the exaggeration is most marked for visitors to elderly mentally infirm patients where the mean distance and mean cost of strategy S were both 97% of their values for strategy R, whereas the mean hospital distance of S was only 78% that of R.

Although the average hospital distance may exaggerate the differences between strategies for visitors and for trips that are subject to suppression by distance, its similarity with the patient travel indices examined make it a useful approximation for situations when it would be impracticable to use a more elaborate evaluation method. Simplicity and ease of calculation from readily accessible census information are its main advantages, and these must be weighed against the fact that it is only a rule of thumb approximation for more complex measures that have more meaning. The models described here and the average hospital distance measure are best seen not as alternatives but as two widely separated points on a continuum. A large number of possible methods lie in between the two (and, indeed, beyond the level of complexity of our models). The average hospital distance could, for example, be used in conjunction with patient numbers, mode of transport and cost assumptions to provide an approximate comparison of community and health service costs under various conditions. Average hospital distance could be made a better measure of the average journeys of out-patients and visitors to preconvalescent patients by incorporating suppression by distance assumptions such as the ones used in this study. In a district containing distinct geographical variations in population composition there would be a strong case for weighting the population of each parish or town by its age/sex composition, and so on. A range of approximations are available to suit the requirements and resources of different users.

SUMMARY

The community hospital functions investigated from the point of view of
travel for patients and visitors were out-patient clinics and units for
preconvalescent, geriatric and elderly mentally infirm in-patients.
Nine different strategies were investigated to accommodate 33,000 out-
patient attendances per year, ranging from complete centralisation to a
dispersed network of five smaller clinics. Four strategies for the
location of preconvalescent beds were examined and these involved different combinations of 81 beds in two or three centres. Similarly, four
different strategies involving 290 beds in two or three centres were
tested for geriatric in-patients. The two elderly mentally infirm
strategies represented a simple choice between two and three hospital
units, with 87 beds altogether.

The strategies were evaluated by estimating the most likely patterns
of travel by patients and visitors under each one and summarising some
of the implications. This was achieved by a computer program using
several relationships derived from the surveys of out-patients, in-
patients and visitors. The first step was to establish the most likely
geographical distribution of the various groups of patients and visitors.
The expected modes of transport were then estimated using the distance
of the journey as the main criterion, although for out-patients consideration of car ownership and public transport quality of individual
parishes also helped to determine the breakdown into transport modes.
Relationships between travel distance and cost for different modes of
transport were used to predict likely transport costs under the various
strategies. For out-patients, estimates of journey time were also made.
Costs to the ambulance and hospital car service were not estimated
because of the need for costs per patient mile information, but the
number of patient miles expected to be generated for the health service
by each strategy was recorded.

Of the transport costs likely to be expended annually by patients,
those of out-patients are by far the highest. They range from £15,000
to £35,000 according to strategy if distance is assumed to have no effect
on the referral of out-patients to clinics, and from £14,000 to £22,000
if a distance effect is incorporated. The estimated travel costs of
in-patients are orders of magnitude lower : from £560 to £630 for preconvalescent patients, in the range £240 to £260 for geriatric patients
and less for elderly mentally infirm patients. Clearly, although
individual patients might have high costs, the overall burden on the
community of in-patients travelling to hospital is not heavy. The
overall costs of visiting however, are much more substantial. The 81
preconvalescent beds are estimated to generate between £29,000 and
£38,000 visiting costs annually, according to strategy, while visitors
to occupants of the 290 geriatric beds are expected to spend £47,000 -
£51,000 at 1977 prices. These estimates, rough as they are, should
put the community's monetary costs into perspective against those of the
health service.

Almost without exception, all the indices of performance produce the
same relative order of strategies. Among the out-patients strategies,
the option with only one clinic in King's Lynn adds a further 30-45% to
the value of the mean distance from the clinic, the mean cost to an

out-patient using his own transport and the total number of health
service transport patient-miles, over the same indices for the strategy
representing the present situation of two clinic locations.   By contrast, the same indices for the most dispersed strategy are reduced to
45-60% of their present value.   Of the three-centre strategies, the
one with clinics in King's Lynn, Wisbech and Swaffham is the most
efficient.   The most accessible system of four centres is with clinics
in King's Lynn, Wisbech, Swaffham and Hunstanton, although this is only
marginally better than the strategy which includes Downham Market in
place of Hunstanton.

Of the four preconvalescent strategies tested, the one which postulates a larger unit in King's Lynn and smaller units in Wisbech and
Swaffham is the most accessible in terms of all the indices examined,
with the index levels around 70-80% of their values in the strategy
representing the likely situation in the early 1980s.   Less variation
is evident among the geriatric options, but again the combination of
King's Lynn, Wisbech and Swaffham proves the most efficient.   If the
choice is between most beds in King's Lynn together with only a few in
Wisbech or a more even distribution between the two towns, the measures
of patient and visitor travel indentify the latter as preferable.
Finally, examination of visiting to elderly mentally infirm patients
shows that the advantages of an extra unit in Swaffham, in addition to
units in King's Lynn and Wisbech, would be minimal.

While the purpose of the exercise is to demonstrate a method for
estimating some of the implications for the community of different
hospital locations, the method used is complex and time-consuming.
Furthermore, while the method does provide consistent measures of the
relative efficiency of the strategies, the absolute measures of cost
and so on rest on too many assumptions to be considered precise.   An
approximation, the "average hospital distance", is suggested as a short
cut method for estimating the relative performances of location strategies.   This index is simple to calculate and it gives a good approximation to the relative values of most, but not all, of the more complex
indices.   It can readily be used to make "quick and dirty" evaluations
of the accessibility of different hospital location strategies or it
can be modified in a number of ways to produce more refined estimates.

7 Conclusions

Our study has been largely based on work in one rural health district.
This raises the question of the applicability of our findings to other
parts of the country. Some findings are undoubtedly quite specific
to the study area. Most of the results in the last chapter, for
example, were concerned with unique patterns of hospital location and
population distribution in the King's Lynn Health District and have no
direct application elsewhere, although it did prove possible to extract
some general conclusions from the specific results. In other chapters
the results reported may also have been affected by the special
characteristics of the study area. The King's Lynn District currently
has poorer hospital facilities, poorer public transport services and
higher car ownership levels than many other rural areas, so certain
findings must be interpreted in this light. Some findings appear to
be less related to the particular features of the King's Lynn District
and are likely to have greater generality. In the pages that follow
we summarise the main conclusions of the study and comment on their
applicability.

Journeys to hospital

The surveys of out-patients and visitors showed that journeys to
hospital were heavily dependent on the private car. Most car users
travelled to hospital in their own car but a considerable number relied
on lifts in someone else's car. For short trips many out-patients and
visitors walked. Public transport was not widely used even by people
without a car. These results reflect the high car ownership levels
and poor bus services of the study district and therefore may not be
typical of rural areas in other parts of the country at the present
time. As car ownership continues to increase and rural bus services
to decline, other districts will increasingly come to resemble the one
studied.

For the majority the costs of each journey to hospital were not great.
Most return trips cost less than £1, although some people did pay more.
For them, and for those making frequent journeys, travel to hospital is
likely to involve significant expenditure.

Many out-patients needed to make special arrangements when they
attended clinics but the need to do this was not related to how far they
had to travel. We conclude that making clinics more accessible would
be unlikely to reduce the need to make special arrangements. However,
the length of time the patient is away from home would inevitably be
related to the location of clinics, and there was also evidence that
the need to be accompanied by another person was greater for longer
journeys. We have no reason to suppose that these findings are limited
to the study district.

The hospitals analysed had very different catchment areas for their in-patients. The majority of visitors lived in the same parish as the patient they had come to visit and therefore their catchment areas corresponded closely to those for in-patients. Many of the visitors to the hospitals serving a wide area did not regularly visit the town the hospital is in. The hospitals with restricted catchment areas had more visitors who were used to visiting the town regularly. They therefore had visiting patterns which conformed more with the day to day life of the community than the hospitals serving a wider area, a conclusion we expect to be valid elsewhere.

The results of the community survey showed that the difficulty of travel to visit patients in hospital was an important source of dissatisfaction. This was particularly so in the remoter villages and for those people likely to have low personal mobility. The community survey also suggested that people (particularly the less mobile) in the remoter villages were less likely to have undertaken such visits. This therefore suggests the possibility that the frequency of visiting is controlled by the accessibility of the hospital. Our visitor surveys showed that for preconvalescent patients both the distance from their homes and the length of time they had been in hospital were important influences on visiting rates. Geriatric patients had fewer visitors, and length of stay (not distance) was the main influence on visiting rates. For elderly mentally infirm patients visiting rates were so low that neither length of stay nor distance had any effect. Our general conclusion is therefore that if the establishment of community hospitals decreased the average distances to patients homes this would tend to increase the number of visitors received by preconvalescent patients but would have no effect on visiting rates to geriatric or elderly mentally infirm patients.

If distance affects visiting rates for some patients, does it also affect the likelihood of using the hospital service as an in-patient or out-patient? The community survey did provide some indications that people in the relatively remote villages were less likely to have been in-patients or out-patients than those living in more accessible villages. The survey of out-patients also revealed that the clinics were used more by those living near to them. However, a study of Hospital Activity Analysis information on in-patient discharges showed no tendency for the remoter rural areas to provide fewer patients, but we do not regard this data source as reliable. Our conclusion is that for out-patients - although possibly not for in-patients - the geographical distribution of hospital services influences the rates of use of hospital services.

The need for community hospitals

If hospitals are used more by those living near to them, people in areas more remote from the hospitals, particularly the less mobile members of the community, will benefit least from them. By increasing the accessibility of hospital services community hospitals would be likely to spread benefits more widely through the community. This would undoubtedly be beneficial to some of the people in the remoter parts of the district but it would also have the effect of increasing the demands placed upon hospital services.

Several items of evidence from our surveys of general practitioners, hospital doctors and the general public suggested that community hospitals might be able to meet needs in ways that are superior to the existing hospital services of the study area. Our research showed that the general practitioners of the King's Lynn District were dissatisfied with the arrangements for admitting elderly chronic patients into hospital, arrangements for admissions on social grounds and the information received about patients whilst they were in hospital. That is, they regarded as inadequate those aspects of the hospital service most likely to be improved by the development of community hospitals. To some extent this may reflect a dissatisfaction with the total amount of hospital provision for these groups of patients. If this is the case, unless community hospitals actually added to the total number of beds available there is no guarantee that they would remove the source of this dissatisfaction. However, the fact that the rural general practitioners in our survey were considerably more dissatisfied than their urban counterparts suggests that remoteness from hospitals is a problem, and one that might well be alleviated by the development of community hospitals. It should be emphasised that this conclusion might not apply in other districts where the current provision of services is different from that in the study district.

Our surveys also produced more general findings. Among both general practitioners and hospital doctors there was widespread agreement that small local hospitals seem less formal and forbidding to patients than larger hospitals, and that patients derive benefits from being cared for in hospitals close to their home. The community survey showed that the general public would be likely to endorse these opinions. Thus, there is strong evidence of the existence of opinions favourable to the development of community hospitals. The smallness and accessibility of such hospitals would both be seen as positive features which for some patients would represent an improvement over the existing hospital services of the district.

The functions of community hospitals

Amongst both hospital doctors and general practitioners our surveys revealed general agreement with the DHSS guidelines on functions. It was widely accepted that general practitioners should be responsible for the medical care of patients but that consultants should hold outpatient clinics in community hospitals. Although there was more disagreement on these issues, a majority also thought that no maternity delivery facilities should be provided and that only simple surgical procedures would be appropriate to community hospitals. The suitability of the elderly mentally infirm for treatment in community hospitals was a very much more contentious issue. Amongst the small majority who stated that these patients should not be treated in community hospitals there were comments that they would be disruptive to other patients, that they need special nursing care and that staffing a hospital containing such patients would be difficult. The fact that many nurses and rehabilitative staff said they were not interested in working with the elderly mentally ill does indeed suggest that staffing might be a problem. It may well be that further consideration needs to be given to the policy of treating the elderly mentally infirm in community hospitals, not only within the study district but in all rural districts.

With the exception of the elderly mentally infirm there was considerable agreement amongst doctors as to the types of patients suitable for community hospitals.   However, the results of the survey of hospital doctors suggested that consultants in the King's Lynn District would be very reluctant to release patients to community hospitals.   This view must be at least partly a reflection of the low number of hospital beds per thousand population in the study district. Without consultant supervision we estimate that only about 30 would be released and with such supervision the number would rise to about 150.   These figures compare with a 1981 norm for the district of up to 260 community hospital beds.   It seems that for the most part community hospitals in districts like the one studied will have to serve a different type of patient than those currently in hospital. That a demand for hospital beds for such patients exists has already been suggested by the results of our survey of general practitioners. The difficulty is in reconciling the view that such patients should be treated in community hospitals with the DHSS's requirement that community hospitals should not add to the total number of hospital beds in a district.   In the long term the rehabilitative role of community hospitals might succeed in extending the active life of people in the community and hence reduce the demands on the hospital service.   In the shorter term there are considerable doubts as to whether the major role of community hospitals will be to relieve pressure on the district general hospitals in districts like the King's Lynn District where the pressure is great.   The extension of care to those not currently using the hospital service seems a more likely role for community hospitals. To do this it appears certain that they will require additional resources.

Staffing

Our survey revealed that a very high proportion of the general practitioners in the King's Lynn District would be interested in working in a community hospital.   Thus the prospects of attracting GPs to work in a community hospital appear to be good.   However, the comments of the GPs suggested that in practice their commitment to a community hospital would probably depend on a reduction of their existing workload and on adequate remuneration.

There was also evidence that careful attention would have to be paid to the location of the hospitals.   The willingness of GPs to participate was shown to fall quite markedly with increasing distance to the community hospital.   In many rural areas where GPs are rather thin on the ground some potential hospital locations might be infeasible because there are insufficient GPs within reasonable travelling distance. However, our survey also revealed that doctors in the rural areas were prepared to travel longer distances than their urban counterparts, so this constraint is unlikely to be particularly severe.

In some specialties where sophisticated equipment is necessary out-patient clinics in community hospitals will obviously not be possible. However, the replies of the hospital doctors questioned in the King's Lynn District suggest that perhaps as many as a half of all out-patient attendances could be in a community hospital with only simple facilities. Where the total number of attendances in a specialty is small, the numbers might be insufficient to justify holding a clinic there.

For the larger specialties this constraint is unlikely to be important. Even considering only the four largest specialties concerned, we estimate that about 40 per cent of the total out-patient attendances of the district could be at community hospitals and we expect this estimate to hold good in other health districts. We have also shown that the willingness of consultants to hold decentralised clinics is greatest in the specialties where the largest numbers could be seen. The prospects for out-patient clinics in community hospitals therefore seem good. In recruiting nurses, physiotherapists, occupational therapists and radiographers two of the problems facing community hospitals might be their distinctive mix of patient types and the small size of the hospitals. With the possible exception of elderly mentally infirm patients, our survey suggests that the types of patient likely to be found in community hospitals are unlikely to substantially discourage the recruitment of nurses. Nor is the smallness of community hospitals likely to be a handicap in the recruitment of nurses. Physiotherapists, occupational therapists and radiographers were markedly less enthusiastic than the nurses about the mix of patients, suggesting that this might prove to be more of a problem in the recruitment of these groups of staff. They were also more likely to express a preference for working in a large hospital. If there are difficulties in recruiting such staff the function of the community hospital as a supportive and rehabilitative centre might well be jeopardised.

One of the arguments in favour of community hospitals is that they could make use of local pools of trained staff who are not prepared to travel long distances to work in a district general hospital. We consider that this is unlikely to be the case. Our surveys suggest that trained staff are a very mobile group. There is also evidence from a national study that factors such as marriage and children (not distance) are the main factors which keep trained staff out of work. Our conclusion is therefore that the development of community hospitals in the King's Lynn District could not be based on attracting back to work a substantial number of trained staff in the district not currently working. It is more likely that community hospitals would compete for staff with other hospitals. We expect this to be true in all but the most severely inaccessible parts of the country.

Methods for the testing of strategies

Many of our findings were incorporated into a model for estimating some of the implications of different hospital locations. Like the study as a whole, this model concentrates on some of the issues on which health service planners are likely to have least information. We give particular emphasis to the accessibility of hospitals to the general public. This is not meant to imply that these are the only factors that need to be considered. The costs of different strategies and the medical benefits associated with each are obviously of vital importance. However, health service planners and the medical profession are in a much better position than we are to estimate these things. Furthermore, studies such as those by Rickard (1976) and by Bennett (1974) provide extensive information on such issues, to which we would be able to add little. For example, Rickard shows that a hospital with only 35 beds can be just as cheap to run (per bed) as a hospital of twice that size. Thus community hospitals considerably smaller than the 50 to 150 bed range suggested by the DHSS appear to be feasible on cost grounds. In an evaluation of different strategies for the development of community hospitals factors such as these would need to be considered alongside the accessibility questions dealt with by our model.

The method which was developed applied several relationships discovered in the surveys of visitors, out-patients and in-patients to census data. For a variety of hospital location strategies, the origins of trips, the distances likely to be covered, the modes of transport that would be used and the costs and times of trips were predicted. We found that travel costs for in-patients were very low, whereas the costs for out-patients and visitors were much greater. When different strategies were compared there was shown to be considerable scope for reducing the transport costs of out-patients and visitors. However, there was a general tendency for the improvements in accessibility to be less as the number of centres increased. These general conclusions are not thought to be dependent on the particular district and strategies studied.

Even on accessibility issues the model, as developed, is not comprehensive, since it predicts the travel costs only of out-patients, in-patients and visitors. The travel costs of day patients or of consultants travelling to out-patient clinics in community hospitals were not considered. However, if estimates of such costs were required they could be derived in a similar way to the costs that are predicted by the model. In this way the method can be adapted to meet particular requirements.

Inevitably the model involved a large number of assumptions, some of which might be inaccurate. It is open to any user of such a method to refine the assumptions which appear to be unacceptable. However, it should be recognised that even this first attempt at a model was quite complex and involved many thousands of calculations, making the use of a computer a virtual necessity. It appeared to us that rather than requiring a more complicated model, many users might want a simpler method for evaluating different hospital location strategies. We suggested the use of an easily calculated index which we call the "average hospital distance". This was shown to approximate quite closely to the relative values of most of the indices produced by the more complex model. It could readily be used in the exploratory stages of evaluation, and with a few modifications might meet most requirements of users.

Conclusion

By exploring the issues, we have attempted to provide evidence that is helpful to those planning the future of small hospitals in rural areas. Some of the results of this study are inevitably peculiar to the district we chose to investigate but we believe that other of our findings have more general applicability. Even where our particular results might not be applicable to another area, our methods of gathering information might. Compared with the time and costs involved in implementing hospital plans the information in this book was gathered quickly and cheaply. Where such information is necessary for the planning of hospital services it should be possible to collect it.

The planner has a responsibility to consider not only the costs of different strategies to the health service but also various costs to patients, their visitors and to the public at large. The problem is that accounting procedures for internal costs are well developed whereas the estimation of community costs is often at a much more rudimentary level. Inevitably there is a risk that community costs will receive insufficient attention. One of the main messages of this book is that this does not need to be the case. We have tried to show that such costs can be estimated and incorporated into evaluation methods. It is to be hoped that the result will be a pattern of hospital services that better meets the needs of the community.

Appendices

POSTAL SURVEY OF HOSPITAL DOCTORS

Your replies to this questionnaire will be treated in confidence. The results
will be presented only in aggregated form so the identification of individuals
will not be possible. If you do not wish to answer some of the questions, please
fill in the parts you feel able to and return the questionnaire - it will still
be valuable to us.

1. Name . . . .

2. Please indicate your age group

under 30	30-39	40-49	50-59	60 and over
☐	☐	☐	☐	☐

3. Higher qualifications . . . .

VIEWS ON COMMUNITY HOSPITAL POLICY

Introduction

In 1974, the Department of Health and Social Security published its 'Community
Hospitals' policy (an extract from the Circular has been enclosed for your
information). In summary, the policy is to establish a network of small local
hospitals which will complement the district general hospital by providing care
for patients who do not need the specialised facilities of a large hospital yet
who cannot be properly cared for at home. The 'community hospitals' are viewed
as an extension of primary care, being staffed by general practitioners and
possessing the facilities to which general practitioners would normally have access.
A health centre or group practice would often be attached to the hospital,
outpatient clinics would be held there and the hospital would have rehabilitative
facilities for day patients. Each community hospital is expected to have 50-150
beds (which is larger than many existing small hospitals). About two thirds of
the beds are expected to be taken by elderly patients. The remaining third will
be for general medical and surgical patients usually on their way to or from
treatment in a district general hospital, and also for patients who are admitted
for short stays to relieve families.

4. By circling the appropriate number, please indicate your response to each
    statement using the following scale:

Strongly Agree	Agree	Neither Agree nor Disagree	Disagree	Strongly Disagree
1	2	3	4	5

	Strongly agree		Neither		Strongly Disagree	Please write any comments here
Small local hospitals seem less formal and forbidding to patients than larger hospitals.	1	2	3	4	5	
Patients derive benefit from care in hospitals near their homes where they can easily be visited and maintain their links with the community.	1	2	3	4	5	

	Strongly agree		Neither		Strongly disagree	Please write any comments here

The fear of hospitals felt by some elderly patients is often strong enough to impair the beneficial effects of hospital care.   1   2   3   4   5

Day to day medical care both of inpatients and day patients in small local hospitals should be provided by GPs.   1   2   3   4   5

Surgical procedures undertaken in small local hospitals should not extend beyond those which GPs would expect to perform in their own practice premises or in a health centre.   1   2   3   4   5

No delivery (maternity) facilities should be provided in small local hospitals.   1   2   3   4   5

Consultants should hold out-patients clinics at small local hospitals whenever possible.   1   2   3   4   5

Greater efforts should be made to admit elderly patients to hospital for short rather than long stays.   1   2   3   4   5

District nurses should also nurse patients in small local hospitals.   1   2   3   4   5

In places where there is a small nospital, the local group practice premises should be attached or in its grounds.   1   2   3   4   5

No emergency or accident cases should be treated in a small local hospital other than those which would normally be dealt with in a GPs surgery.   1   2   3   4   5

Elderly patients with dementia should be looked after in small local hospitals which also have other types of patients.   1   2   3   4   5

5. <u>Inpatients in your specialty.</u>

What proportion of the inpatients for whom you have responsibility at the present time could be adequately cared for in a small local hospital by a GP <u>without direct consultant supervision</u>? Please tick the category which most nearly applies;

none   10% or   20%   30%   40%   50%   60%   70%   80%   90%   100%
       less

☐   ☐   ☐   ☐   ☐   ☐   ☐   ☐   ☐   ☐   ☐

<u>Are any of these patients:</u>   tick those which apply

     social admissions...................................
     terminal admissions................................
     *preconvalescents..................................
     geriatric patients.................................
     geriatric patients with dementia..................
     patients undergoing rehabilitation................
     other (please specify)
     ....

6. What additional proportion of the inpatients for whom you have responsibility could be adequately cared for in a small local hospital by a GP but <u>under the direct supervision of a consultant</u>?
(Do not include any patients referred to in the previous question).
Please tick the category that most nearly applies;

none   10% or   20%   30%   40%   50%   60%   70%   80%   90%   100%
       less

☐   ☐   ☐   ☐   ☐   ☐   ☐   ☐   ☐   ☐   ☐

<u>Are any of these patients:</u>   tick those which apply

     social admissions...................................
     terminal admissions................................
     *preconvalescents..................................
     geriatric patients.................................
     geriatric patients with dementia..................
     patients undergoing rehabilitation................
     other (please specify) ....
     ....

7. <u>Outpatients clinics in your specialty in the King's Lynn Health District</u>

Do you attend any outpatients clinics?   yes ☐   no ☐   (IF NO GO TO QUESTION 11)

If yes:

Hospital at which clinic is held	Specialty or department	Number of sessions that you attend each month

*Patients who have already received elsewhere the most intensive part of their treatment, but who still require active nursing care and medical supervision.

4.

8. If a community hospital had the following facilities:

    consulting room
    examination room
    clinical test room
    reception office
    patient's waiting room
    straight X-ray facility
    specimen collection service
    pharmaceutical service
    nursing and secretarial support

    a. What proportion of your outpatients who are first attendances
        could you see satisfactorily?   (please tick one)

none	10% or less	20%	30%	40%	50%	60%	70%	80%	90%	100%
☐	☐	☐	☐	☐	☐	☐	☐	☐	☐	☐

    b. What proportion of your outpatients who are re-attendances could you
        see satisfactorily?   (please tick one)

none	10% or less	20%	30%	40%	50%	60%	70%	80%	90%	100%
☐	☐	☐	☐	☐	☐	☐	☐	☐	☐	☐

    List any additional facilities which would substantially increase these
    proportions ....
    ....

9. What are the main advantages and disadvantages from your point of view
    of holding outpatients clinics in smaller hospitals away from the
    general hospital?

            advantages   disadvantages

    ....

    ....

    ....

    ....

    ....

10. On balance do you agree with the principle of holding such decentralised
    clinics for your specialty?   (please tick one)

        yes ☐   no ☐   don't know ☐

11. Have you any general comments about the Community Hospital Policy?

THANK YOU FOR YOUR HELP

1.

University of East Anglia

Community Hospital Planning Study

Survey of General Practitioners in the King's Lynn Health District.

Your replies to this questionnaire will be treated in confidence. The results will be presented only in aggregated form so the identification of individuals will not be possible. If you do not wish to answer some of the questions, please fill in the parts you feel able to and return the questionnaire - it will still be valuable to us.

(A)   PERSONAL INFORMATION

1.   Sex (please tick) ....M ☐   F ☐

2.   Age (please tick)   Under 30   30-39   40-49   50-59   60 and over
                            ☐   ☐   ☐   ☐   ☐

3.   What higher qualifications do you possess? ....
     ....

4.   How long have you been a GP in your present practice?............☐ years.

5.   Are you in partnership? (please tick)   Yes ☐   No ☐
     If you are in partnership, please state:

                                          Full-time   Part-time

        Number of principals ....   _____   _____

        Number of assistants ....   _____   _____

        Number of vacancies ....   _____   _____

6.   How many ancillary staff in the following categories work in your practice? (in your group practice, if in partnership):

	Attached to practice		Employed by practice	
	Full-time	Part-time	Full-time	Part-time
Secretary/receptionist........	_____	_____	_____	_____
Nurse	_____	_____	_____	_____
Midwife	_____	_____	_____	_____
Health visitor..............	_____	_____	_____	_____

7.   Are your main surgery premises purpose-built? ....Yes ☐   No ☐

8.   Have you held any full-time post-registration hospital appointments for 6 months or more?   Yes ☐   No ☐

     If yes, please state specialty or specialties ....

     What was the most senior level of your appointment? (please tick)

Senior House Officer   Registrar   Senior Registrar   Medical Assistant   Other

        ☐   ☐   ☐   ☐   ☐

9. How many patients are there on your personal NHS list? (If you are in partnership and have no personal list, what is the average list size for each GP in your practice? Please tick:

0-999	1000-1499	1500 -1999	2000-2499	2500-2999	3000-3499	3500-3999	4000 and above
☐	☐	☐	☐	☐	☐	☐	☐

10. Do you currently hold any hospital posts (eg. clinical assistantship)? Yes ☐
    (Please tick)   No ☐

    If yes, Appointment _____

    Number of sessions per week _____

11. Can you admit your patients to a hospital bed under your own care? (Please tick)

    (a) Maternity ....Yes ☐   No ☐

    (b) Other ....Yes ☐   No ☐

(B) VIEWS ON YOUR PRESENT WORK

12. In your own experience in this district, how would you describe the adequacy of the following? (please tick):

	Adequate	Inadequate	Most Inadequate	Please write any comments here
(a) Arrangements for admitting elderly acute patients into hospital				
(b) Arrangements for admitting elderly chronic patients into hospital				
(c) Arrangements for admitting patients to hospital on social grounds.............				
(d) The information you receive from hospital concerning the investigation, treatment and progress of your patients whilst they are in hospital.				
(e) The speed with which you receive information from the hospital after discharge of your patients..............				
(f) The information you receive from the hospital following a visit to an outpatient clinic by one of your patients...................				

13. Are there any groups of patients-or types of cases-that you have particular difficulty in getting admitted to hospital?   Yes ☐   No ☐

If yes, please specify ....

....

14. What do you feel about the adequacy of the following services in your locality? (please tick). If you have contacted any of them on behalf of a patient during the last month, please also tick in right hand column.

	Adequate	Inadequate	Most Inadequate	Recent Contact	Please write any comments here
(a) District nurses.......					
(b) Physiotherapists......					
(c) Health visitors.......					
(d) Chiropodists..........					
(e) Social workers........					
(f) Home helps............					
(g) Meals on wheels.......					
(h) Voluntary associations.........					

15. Assuming that you are able to make the necessary time available, in what direction would you wish to develop interests in the future? (please tick)

	Very Interested	Interested	Not Interested
(a) Working solely as a family doctor in General Practice..........			
(b) Pursuit of a special clinical interest by hospital appointment (if interested, please state specialty of choice)			
(c) Early care of hospital inpatients after surgery......................			
(d) Care of geriatric patients in hospital beds.....................			
(e) Care of patients in hospital who require admission on social grounds..........................			
(f) Care of hospital day patients.......			
(g) Work in pre-school and school health clinics.....................			
(h) Other-please specify			

(C)   VIEWS ON COMMUNITY HOSPITAL POLICY

Introduction

In 1974, the Department of Health and Social Security published its 'Community
Hospitals' policy (an extract from the Circular has been enclosed for your
information).   In summary, the policy is to establish a network of small
local hospitals which will complement the district general hospital by
providing care for patients who do not need the specialised facilities of a
large hospital yet who cannot be properly cared for at home.   These
'community hospitals' are viewed as an extension of primary care, being
staffed by general practitioners and possessing the facilities to which
general practitioners would normally have access.   A health centre or group
practice would often be attached to the hospital, outpatient clinics would
be held there and the hospital would have rehabilitative facilities for day
patients.   Each community hospital is expected to have 50-150 beds (which
is larger than many existing small hospitals).   About two thirds of the beds
are expected to be taken by elderly patients.   The remaining third will
be for general medical and surgical patients usually on their way to or from
treatment in a district general hospital, and also for patients who are
admitted for short stays to relieve families.

16.   By circling the appropriate number, please indicate your response to
       each statement using the following scale:

Strongly agree	Agree	Neither agree nor disagree	Disagree	Strongly disagree
1	2	3	4	5

	Strongly agree		Neither		Strongly disagree	Please write any comments here
Small local hospitals seem less formal and forbidding to patients than larger hospitals.	1	2	3	4	5	
Patients derive benefit from care in hospitals near their homes where they can easily be visited and maintain their links with the community.	1	2	3	4	5	
The fear of hospitals felt by some elderly patients is often strong enough to impair the beneficial effects of hospital care.	1	2	3	4	5	
Day to day medical care both of inpatients and day patients in small local hospitals should be provided by GPs.	1	2	3	4	5	

	Strongly agree		Neither		Strongly disagree

Please write any comments here

Surgical procedures undertaken in small local hospitals should not extend beyond those which GPs would expect to perform in their own practice premises or in a health centre.
1   2   3   4   5

No delivery (maternity) facilities should be provided in small local hospitals.
1   2   3   4   5

Consultants should hold out-patients clinics at small local hospitals whenever possible.
1   2   3   4   5

Greater efforts should be made to admit elderly patients to hospital for short rather than long stays.
1   2   3   4   5

District nurses should also nurse patients in small local hospitals.
1   2   3   4   5

In places where there is a small hospital, the local group practice premises should be attached or in its grounds.
1   2   3   4   5

No emergency or accident cases should be treated in a small local hospital other than those which would normally be dealt with in a GPs surgery.
1   2   3   4   5

Elderly patients with dementia should be looked after in small local hospitals which also have other types of patients.
1   2   3   4   5

17.   In principle, do you feel that you would like to participate in a Community Hospital?   (please tick)

I definitely would wish to participate........................

I may wish to participate....................................

I am unlikely to wish to participate.........................

I definitely would not wish to participate...................

I don't know...

Other (please specify)_____

18. How interested would you be in working in a Community Hospital at the following distances from your home?   (please tick)

	Very Interested	Interested	Not Interested
(a) 0 - 5 miles			
(b) 5 - 10 miles			
(c) Over 10 miles			

19. If working in a Community Hospital involved periods of being on call for a minor accident service (say once every two weeks), how interested would you be in working in a Community Hospital at the following distances from your home?   (please tick)

	Very Interested	Interested	Not Interested
(a) 0 - 5 miles			
(b) 5 - 10 miles			
(c) Over 10 miles			

20. Have you any general comments about the Community Hospital policy?

THANK YOU FOR YOUR HELP.

UNIVERSITY OF EAST ANGLIA

COMMUNITY HOSPITAL PLANNING STUDY

SURVEY OF HOSPITAL NURSES, PHYSIOTHERAPISTS
OCCUPATIONAL THERAPISTS AND RADIOGRAPHERS

1. What is your present occupation? Please tick one of the following

        Nurse .... ☐

        Physiotherapist.................... ☐

        Occupational therapist .... ☐

        Radiographer...................... ☐

        Other(please specify) _____

    What is your present grade? _____

2. What professional qualifications do you have?

        Please specify_____

        _____

3. Are you working full-time or part-time at present? Please tick one of
the following.

        Full-time ☐   Part-time ☐

4. Which town or village do you live in? (If you do not live in a town
or village, what is the town or village nearest you home?)

        Name of town or village_____

5. How do you usually travel to work? (please tick one of the following,
the one you come furthest on).

        driving the household car............................. ☐

        as a passenger in the household car .... ☐

        as a passenger in a car not owned by your............ ☐
        household, without any payment

        as a passenger in a car not owned by your
        household, with some contribution toward the cost...... ☐

        walking or by bicycle .... ☐

        public bus or train .... ☐

        transport organised by the hospital.................. ☐

        motorcycle or moped.................................. ☐

        no journey involved .... ☐

        other .... ☐

6. How long does it usually take to travel to work? Please circle
   the nearest time:

   <u>Minutes</u>   5   10   15   20   25   30   35   40   45   50   55   60

                    (over 60 minutes, please specify time:) [   ]

7. If you travel by bus or train what is the cost of the single fare for
   one person?

                    Cost [£   :   p   ]

8. Do you usually travel to <u>and</u> from work in the peak period?
   (i.e. 7.30-9 a.m. and 4-6.30 p.m.)

                    Yes [ ]   No [ ]

9. When you first started work in this hospital which <u>one</u> of the following
   statements applied to you? (please tick one)

   You had been living in the area previously (for at least
   6 months) .... [ ]

   You moved into the area primarily to be able to work in
   <u>this</u> hospital.. [ ]

   You moved into the area primarily to look for employment in
   <u>any</u> hospital in the vicinity..................................... [ ]

   You moved into the area primarily for another reason (e.g.
   husband's or wife's work, family reasons, other reasons)......... [ ]

10. Have you worked in any of the following? (please tick those
    which apply)
                    A hospital with less than 50 beds................ [ ]
                    A hospital with 50-99 beds....................... [ ]
                    A hospital with 100-300 beds..................... [ ]
                    A hospital with more than 300 beds............... [ ]

11. How do you feel about working with the following patient-types?
                    (please tick one box for each patient type)

Patient types	Very Interested	Interested	Not Interested	Don't know or not applicable
Geriatric				
*Pre-convalescent				
Physically handicapped				
Elderly patients suffering from dementia				
Terminal				

* Patients who have already received elsewhere the most intensive part of
  their treatment, but who still require active nursing care and medical
  supervision.

12. How important are the following for your job satisfaction?
    (please tick one box for each statement)

	For my job satisfaction		
	Very Important	Important	Not Important
(a) A wide variety of types of patients to care for.			
(b) Being able to get to know patients personally.			
(c) Flexibility and variety in work.			
(d) Plenty of information on the home circumstances of patients.			
(e) A lot of contact with hospital doctors.			
(f) A lot of contact with the General Practitioners of patients.			
(g) A lot of contact with the district nurses who will care for discharged patients.			
(h) Use of and experience with the most modern equipment.			
(i) Working with experienced and skilled hospital staff.			
(j) Work which makes full use of training and experience.			
(k) Opportunities to increase training and experience.			
(l) Personal preferences for desirable working hours and time off taken into account.			
(m) The social life of the hospital.			
(n) Friendly relationships with all hospital staff with whom you work regularly.			
(o) Each member of the hospital staff feeling that his/her contribution is valued by other members of the hospital staff.			
(p) The opportunity to live in.			

13. In your opinion, which of the following are found more often in large hospitals (say over 300 beds), which are found more often in small hospitals (say less than 50 beds) and which are equally present or absent in all sizes of hospitals? Please tick one box for each statement.

		More often found in LARGE hospitals	Not related to size of hospital	More often found in SMALL hospital
(a)	A wide variety of types of patients to care for.			
(b)	Being able to get to know patients personally.			
(c)	Flexibility and variety in work.			
(d)	Plenty of information on the home circumstances of patients.			
(e)	A lot of contact with hospital doctors.			
(f)	A lot of contact with the General Practitioners of patients.			
(g)	A lot of contact with the district nurses who will care for discharged patients.			
(h)	Use of and experience with the most modern equipment.			
(i)	Working with experienced and skilled hospital staff.			
(j)	Work which makes full use of training and experience.			
(k)	Opportunities to increase training and experience.			
(l)	Personal preferences for desirable working hours and time off taken into account.			
(m)	The social life of the hospital.			
(n)	Friendly relationships with all hospital staff with whom you work regularly.			
(o)	Each member of the hospital staff feeling that his/her contribution is valued by other members of the hospital staff.			
(p)	The opportunity to live in.			

14. Which size of hospital would you prefer to work in?
    Please tick one of the following.

    A hospital with less than 50 beds.. ☐

    A hospital with 50-99 beds........ ☐

    A hospital with 100-300 beds...... ☐

    A hospital with more than 300 beds. ☐

    No particular preference.......... ☐

15. What age group are you in?   Please tick one of the following:

    under 20   20 - 29   30 - 39   40 - 49   50 - 59   60 and over
      ☐   ☐   ☐   ☐   ☐   ☐

16. Please indicate you sex and marital status:

    Female ☐   Single ☐

    Male ☐   Married ☐

                                  Widowed or ☐
                                  Divorced

                    THANK YOU FOR YOUR HELP
                    _____

SURVEY OF OUTPATIENTS

We are trying to find out about your journey to this outpatient clinic. It would
help us greatly if each PATIENT at today's clinic could fill in this short questionnaire.
People accompanying patients may complete the form on behalf of the patient.
Individual replies will be treated in confidence.

Dr. R.M. Haynes,
Community Hospital Planning Study,
University of East Anglia.

ALL ANSWERS SHOULD REFER TO THE PATIENT

1. Have you ever been to this outpatients clinic before (because of the same complaint)?

   (Please tick)   YES☐   NO☐

2. How did you get to the hospital today? (please tick one of the following - the one
   you travelled furthest on)

using the hospital car service.....................☐   in an ambulance................☐
driving the household car..........................☐   on a motorcycle or moped.......☐
as a passenger in your household's car............☐   on foot or bicycle.............☐
as a passenger in a car owned by a relative,   by public bus or train.........☐
   friend or neighbour (without payment)..........☐   in a taxi......................☐
as a passenger in a car owned by a relative,friend   by other means.................☐
   or neighbour (with some contribution to costs)..☐

3. Do you intend to leave by the same means?(please tick)   YES☐   NO☐

   If you came by bus or train, what was the cost
   of the single fare for one person?   £ : P

4. Where did you come to the hospital from? (please tick)   HOME☐ WORK☐ OTHER☐

   Where is this?   (name of town or village)   _____

   Did you come straight from there? (please tick) ....YES☐   NO☐

   How long did it take? .... time [   ]

5. Where are you going when you leave
   the hospital? (please tick)..................... HOME☐ WORK☐ OTHER☐

   Where is this? (name of town or village)   _____

6. Other than coming to the hospital which of the following will you do, or have you
   done, in **WISBECH** today?

   nothing else..............☐   go to work...................☐
   shopping..................☐   go to bank...................☐
   take children to school or   visit post office............☐
      pick them up from school.☐   other (please write in)
                                      _____

   Would you have needed to come to WISBECH anyway?

   (please tick)   YES☐   NO☐

PLEASE TURN OVER

190

7. How often do you visit **WISBECH** other than to come to the hospital? (please tick)

    daily....................☐   2 or 3 times each month....☐
    2 or 3 times each week....☐   monthly....................☐
    weekly....................☐   less often................☐

8. Have you got a current driving licence? (please tick)   YES☐   NO☐

9. How many cars are owned by members of your household?   (please tick)

    no cars   1 car   2 cars   3 or more cars
    ☐   ☐   ☐   ☐

10. How many people came with you to the hospital today?   (please tick)

    nobody   1 person   2 people   3 or more people
    ☐   ☐   ☐   ☐

11. Did you need to make special arrangements at home or work to come to the hospital today? (please tick as many as appropriate)

    no special arrangement made..............................☐
    ask somebody to look after the children..................☐
    take time off work for which you are not paid............☐
    take time off work without loss of pay...................☐
    ask somebody who usually goes out to work to come with you.☐
    ask somebody who usually goes out to work to stay at home..☐
    make any other special arrangements (please write in)

12. Which age group are you in?   (please tick)

    under 15   15-24   25-44   45-64   65-74   over 75
    ☐   ☐   ☐   ☐   ☐   ☐

13. Please indicate your sex   MALE☐   FEMALE☐

THANK YOU VERY MUCH FOR YOUR HELP.

INPATIENT QUESTIONNAIRE

Patient No.		Specialty	Ward	Hospital

1. Could you tell me your name please ? _____

2. How did you get to hospital when you were first admitted ?

   in an ambulance........................ ☐
   using the hospital car service.......... ☐
   driving the household car............... ☐
   as a passenger in your household's car.. ☐
   as a passenger in other car
      (without payment)................ ☐

   as a passenger in other car
      (with payment).......... ☐
   motorcycle/moped.................... ☐
   foot/bicycle....................... ☐
   public bus or train............... ☐
   taxi.............................. ☐

3. When were you first admitted to the ward ?   day   date   month

   length of stay (inc. day of admission)   ☐☐ days

4. Where do you live ? (name of town or village nearest patient's home if she/he
   does not live in town or village?)

   town or village _____   zone code
   county _____   ☐☐

5. How many different people have come to visit you in the last week ? (or since
   admission if patient has not been in hospital for a week)   ☐☐

   How many times did each of these people visit you in the last week ?

   TOTAL VISITS RECEIVED ☐☐

   Were any of your visitors social workers, from a voluntary organisation or
   from the church ?

             YES   NO   (ring one)

   If yes ask   How many separate visits have you had from someone like this in the
                last week ?
                                TOTAL VISITS RECEIVED ☐☐

6. Would you mind telling me which age group you are in ?   (show card and ring one)

       5-14   15-24   25-44   45-64   65-74   75+

7. Are you married, single, widowed or divorced ?

                male   single
                female   widowed/divorced   (ring two)
                                      married

8. Number of visits received during survey   Number of forms attached
                ☐☐   ☐☐

                Thank you very much for being so helpful.

GROUPS OF PEOPLE WHO TRAVELLED TOGETHER ARE ASKED TO COMPLETE ONE FORM ONLY

1. What is the name of the patient you have come to visit ? _____

2. How many people, including yourself, travelled together to visit the patient ?

    (write in number) ☐

3. When did you arrive at the hospital ? (please tick) BEFORE 5 PM ☐   AFTER 5 PM ☐

4. How did your group get to the hospital today? (please tick one of the following -
    the one you came furthest on).

    in a car........................☐   in a taxi......................☐
    on a motorcycle or moped.........☐   on foot or by bicycle..........☐
    by public bus/train..............☐   by other means.................☐

    Will you make the return journey by the same means?   YES ☐   NO ☐

    If you came by bus and/or train, what
    was the cost of the single fare for one person?   £   :   p

5. Which town or village do you live in? (if you do not live in a town or village,
    what is the town or village nearest to your home?)

    (name of town or village) _____

6. Where did you come to the hospital from? (please tick)   HOME ☐ WORK ☐   OTHER ☐

    Where is this? (name of town or village) _____

    Did you come straight from there? (please tick)........... YES ☐   NO ☐

    How long did it take? .... time ☐

7. Where are you going when you leave
       the hospital? (please tick)...................   HOME ☐ WORK ☐   OTHER ☐

    Where is this? (name of town or village) _____

8. Other than coming to the hospital, which of the following things have been done, or
    will be done, by you or those with you in **KING'S LYNN** today? (tick appropriate boxe

    nothing else....................☐   go to work....................☐
    shopping........................☐   go to bank....................☐
    take children to school or   visit the post office.........☐
       pick them up from school......☐   other (please write in)

    _____

    Would you have needed to come to **KING'S LYNN** anyway?

            YES ☐   NO ☐

We would like some information about each individual.   Could you and the people who
travelled with you each fill in one section overleaf.

1. If you came by car, were you........... the driver............................ ☐
   (please tick one) passenger in household car........... ☐
   passenger in another car............. ☐
   none of these........................ ☐

2. How often do you come to **KING'S LYNN** other than to visit the hospital? (please tick)

   daily....................... ☐   2 or 3 times each month............. ☐
   2 or 3 times each week....... ☐   monthly............................. ☐
   weekly..................... ☐   less often.......................... ☐

3. What is your sex? (please tick)   MALE ☐   FEMALE ☐

4. What age group are you in?   under 15   15-24   25-44   45-64   65-74   over 75
   (please tick one)   ☐   ☐   ☐   ☐   ☐   ☐

5. What is your relationship with the patient you have come to visit? (please tick)

   mother, daughter, sister or wife.. ☐   friend/neighbour..................... ☐
   father, son, brother or husband... ☐   social worker, member of voluntary
   other relative................... ☐   body or church...................... ☐

SECOND PERSON

1. If you came by car, were you.......... the driver............................ ☐
   passenger in household car........... ☐
   passenger in another car............. ☐
   none of these........................ ☐

2. How often do you come to **KING'S LYNN** other than to visit the hospital? (tick one)

   daily....................... ☐   2 or 3 times each month............. ☐
   2 or 3 times each week........ ☐   monthly............................. ☐
   weekly..................... ☐   less often.......................... ☐

3. What is your sex? (please tick)   MALE ☐   FEMALE ☐

4. What age group are you in?   under 15   15-24   25-44   45-64   65-74   over 75
   (please tick one)   ☐   ☐   ☐   ☐   ☐   ☐

5. What is your relationship with the patient you have come to visit? (please tick)

   mother, daughter, sister or wife.. ☐   friend/neighbour..................... ☐
   father, son, brother or husband.... ☐   social worker, member of voluntary
   other relative................... ☐   body or church...................... ☐

THIRD PERSON

1. If you came by car, were you........... the driver............................ ☐
   (please tick one) passenger in household car........... ☐
   passenger in another car............. ☐
   none of these........................ ☐

2. How often do you come to **KING'S LYNN** other than to visit the hospital? (tick one)
   daily....................... ☐   2 or 3 times each month............. ☐
   2 or 3 times each week........ ☐   monthly............................. ☐
   weekly..................... ☐   less often.......................... ☐

3. What is your sex? (please tick)   MALE ☐   FEMALE ☐

4. What age group are you in?   under 15   15-24   25-44   45-64   65-74   over 75
   (please tick one)   ☐   ☐   ☐   ☐   ☐   ☐

5. What is your relationship with the patient you have come to visit? (please tick)

   mother, daughter, sister or wife.. ☐   friend/neighbour..................... ☐
   father, son brother or husband.... ☐   social worker, member of voluntary
   other relative................... ☐   body or church...................... ☐

IF MORE THAN THREE VISITORS TRAVELLED TOGETHER, PLEASE ENTER THE ADDITIONAL INFORMATION
ON THE BACK OF ANOTHER FORM.

COMMUNITY SURVEY

Location........................Interviewer ....Interview No.....

Introduction: Good evening, I am sorry to disturb you.   I am from the University
of East Anglia in Norwich and we are finding out people's views about hospitals in
West Norfolk.   Would you please help us by answering a few questions?   It will only
take five minutes.

1. Have you ever been a patient in hospital?......... YES   NO   DK

2. Have you ever been to hospital as an outpatient?... YES   NO   DK

3. Have you ever visited a patient in hospital?....... YES   NO   DK

4. How many visits have you made to patients in
    hospital during the past year?
    (WRITE IN) . . . . visits.   DK

5. Which of these best describes your feelings about the hospitals which serve
    this part of Norfolk?   (SHOW CARD)

    (1) V. SATIS.   (2) SATIS.   (3) NEITHER   (4) DISSATIS.   (5) V. DISSATIS   (6) DK

6. I am going to read you a list of things connected with hospital facilities.
    Please tell me how satisfied or dissatisfied you are with each of the items.
    (SHOW CARD). Even if you have not been a hospital patient yourself, we are still
    interested in your views as a member of the public.

    (1) V. SATIS.   (2) SATIS.   (3) NEITHER   (4) DISSATIS   (5) V.DISSATIS.   (6) DK

    a. The length of time people who need an operation have
        to wait before being admitted to hospital.............. 1 2 3 4 5 6
    b. The rules and regulations for patients in hospital..... 1 2 3 4 5 6
    c. The friendliness of hospitals......................... 1 2 3 4 5 6
    d. The travelling for people who want to visit patients
        in hospital.. 1 2 3 4 5 6
    e. The amount of information given to patients about
        what is wrong with them.............................. 1 2 3 4 5 6
    f. The visiting hours................................... 1 2 3 4 5 6
    g. The travelling time in getting patients to
        hospital in an emergency............................. 1 2 3 4 5 6
    h. Patients being cared for by doctors and nurses
        they have not met before............................. 1 2 3 4 5 6
    i. The travelling for people who have to get to
        hospital clinics..................................... 1 2 3 4 5 6
    j. Is there anything else you are not satisfied with?

        (WRITE IN) ....

7. If you became ill and needed to go into hospital, and you could receive
    exactly the same medical treatment in a large hospital with about 500 patients or
    in a small hospital with about 50 patients, which would you prefer to be in?

            LARGE   SMALL   DK/OTHER

8. Does anybody in your household own a car?   YES   NO

9. Which age group are you in?   (SHOW CARD)

    (1) Under 44   (2) 45-64   (3) 65-74   (4) 75+   DK/REFUSE

10. Sex of respondent   M   F

11. Occupation of head of household (WRITE IN) ....

THANK YOU VERY MUCH

195

Bibliography

Aday, L. and Andersen, R., Development of Indices of Access to Medical Care, Health Administration Press, Ann Arbor, Mich. 1975.

Ashley, J.S.A., "Present State of Statistics from Hospital In-patient Data and their Uses", British Journal of Preventive and Social Medicine, 26, 1972, pp135-147.

Automobile Association Technical Services, Schedule of Estimated Running Costs : April 1977, Automobile Association, Basingstoke 1977.

Bennett, A.E., (ed), Community Hospitals : Progress in Development and Evaluation, Oxford Regional Hospital Board, Oxford 1974.

Berry, R.E., "Returns to Scale in the Production of Hospital Services", Hospital Services Research, Summer 1969.

Brooks, B.M., An Investigation of Factors Affecting the Use of Buses by both Elderly and Ambulant Disabled Persons, British Leyland Truck and Bus Division, 1974.

Carr, W.J. and Feldstein, P.J., "The Relationship of Cost to Hospital Size", Inquiry, June 1967, pp.45-65.

Central Health Services Council, The Functions of the District General Hospital (Bonham-Carter Report), HMSO, London 1969.

Central Statistical Office, Social Trends, No.8, HMSO, London 1977.

Cmnd 6836 Transport Policy, HMSO, London 1977.

Cohen, H.A., "Variations in cost among hospitals of different sizes", Southern Economic Journal, January 1967.

Cooper, L., "The transportation location problem", Operations Research, 20, 1972, pp.94-108.

Cross, K.W. and Turner, R.D. "Factors Affecting the Visiting Pattern of Geriatric Patients in a Rural Area", British Journal of Preventive and Social Medicine, 28, 1974, pp.133-139.

Department of the Environment, Highway Statistics 1973 HMSO, London 1974.

Department of the Environment, National Travel Survey 1972/3 HMSO, London 1976a.

Department of the Environment, Transport Policy : A Consultative Document, HMSO, London 1976b.

Department of Health and Social Security, Community Hospitals : Their Role and Development in the National Health Service HSC(IS)75, HMSO, London 1974.

Department of Health and Social Security, Sharing Resources for Health in England : Report of the Resource Allocation Working Party, HMSO, London 1976.

Department of Health and Social Security, Health and Personal Social Services Statistics for England, HMSO, London 1977a.

Department of Health and Social Security Priorities in the Health and Social Services : The Way Forward, HMSO, London 1977b.

Department of Health and Social Security and Office of Population Censuses and Surveys, Report on Hospital In-patient Enquiry 1972, HMSO, London 1974.

Department of Health and Social Security and Office of Population Censuses and Surveys, Report on Hospital In-patient Enquiry 1973, HMSO, London 1975.

Department of Transport, Transport Statistics Great Britain 1965-1975, HMSO, London 1977.

Department of Transport, Report of the Advisory Committee on Trunk Road Assessment (Leitch Committee), HMSO, London 1978.

East Anglian Regional Health Authority, Annual Patient Statistics 1975, Cambridge 1976.

East Anglian Regional Health Authority, Population Projections 1981, 1986, 1991, Cambridge 1977.

Edwards, D.A., Spatial Variations in Car Ownership in Rural Areas, MSc thesis, Cranfield Institute of Technology, Centre for Transport Studies, September 1977.

Fairhurst, M.H. "The Influence of Public Transport on Car Ownership in London", Journal of Transport Economics and Policy, September 1975.

Feldstein, M.S., Economic Analysis for Health Service Efficiency, North Holland, Amsterdam 1967.

Fishwick, F., "The Influence of Economic Factors on Car Ownership in Great Britain", Paper presented to PTRC Seminar on Urban Traffic Model Research, London 1972.

Hasler, J.C., "The General Practitioner", in A.E. Bennett (ed) Community Hospitals : Progress in Development and Evaluation, Oxford Regional Hospital Board, Oxford 1974.

Hillman, M., Henderson, I. and Whalley, A., Transport Realities and Planning : Policy Studies of Friction and Freedom in Daily Travel, P.E.P., London 1976.

Ministry of Health, A Hospital Plan for England and Wales, Cmnd.1604, HMSO, London 1962.

Moseley, M.J., Harman, R.G., Coles, O.B. and Spencer, M.B., Rural Transport and Accessibility, Volume 1, Centre of East Anglian Studies, University of East Anglia, 1977a.

Moseley, M.J., Harman, R.G., Coles, O.B. and Spencer, M.B., University of East Anglia Rural Transport and Accessibility Study : unpublished data, 1977b.

Norfolk Area Health Authority, Proposals for Hospital Services in the King's Lynn Health District, Norwich 1978.

Norfolk Councy Council, Norfolk Structure Plan, Norwich 1977.

Norman, A., Transport and the Elderly : Problems and Possible Action, National Corporation for the Care of Old People, London 1977.

Registrar General, Statistical Review of England and Wales, 1973, Part I, HMSO, London 1975.

Rhys, D.G. and Buxton, M.J. "Car Ownership and the Rural Transport Problem", The Chartered Institute of Transport Journal, July 1974.

Rickard, J.H., Cost-Effectiveness Analysis of the Oxford Community Hospital Programme, Health Services Evaluation Group, Department of the Regius Professor of Medicine, University of Oxford 1976.

Ro, K., "Determinants of Hospital Costs", Yale Economic Essays, 1968.

Sadler, J. and Whitworth, T., Reserves of Nurses, HMSO, London 1975.

Tanner, T.C., Forecasts of Vehicles and Traffic in Great Britain - 1974 Revision, Dept. of the Environment, Transport and Road Research Laboratory, LR640, Crowthorne 1974.

Index